Introduction to Sectional Anatomy
WORKBOOK and
REVIEW GUIDE

Second Edition

Introduction to Sectional Anatomy
WORKBOOK and
REVIEW GUIDE

Second Edition

Mike E. Madden, PhD, RT(R) (CT) (MR)

Director
Medical Diagnostic Imaging Programs
Fort Hays State University
Hays, Kansas

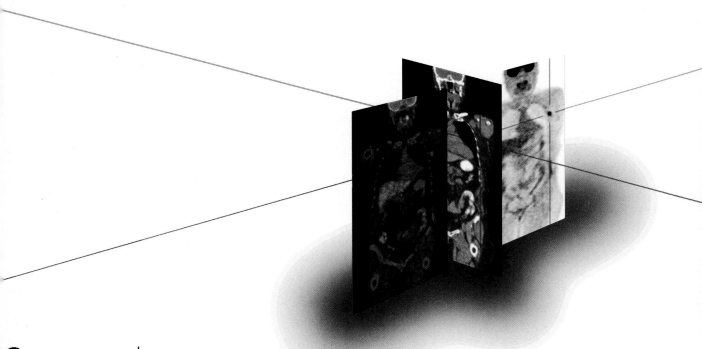

Wolters Kluwer | Lippincott Williams & Wilkins
Health
Philadelphia • Baltimore • New York • London
Buenos Aires • Hong Kong • Sydney • Tokyo

Acquisitions Editor: Peter Sabatini
Managing Editor: Andrea M. Klingler
Marketing Manager: Allison Noplock
Production Editor: Kevin P. Johnson
Designer: Teresa Mallon
Compositor: Aptara, Inc.

Second Edition

DISCLAIMER

Care has been taken to confirm the accuracy of the information present and to describe generally accepted practices. However, the authors, editors, and publisher are not responsible for errors or omissions or for any consequences from application of the information in this book and make no warranty, expressed or implied, with respect to the currency, completeness, or accuracy of the contents of the publication. Application of this information in a particular situation remains the professional responsibility of the practitioner; the clinical treatments described and recommended may not be considered absolute and universal recommendations.

The authors, editors, and publisher have exerted every effort to ensure that drug selection and dosage set forth in this text are in accordance with the current recommendations and practice at the time of publication. However, in view of ongoing research, changes in government regulations, and the constant flow of information relating to drug therapy and drug reactions, the reader is urged to check the package insert for each drug for any change in indications and dosage and for added warnings and precautions. This is particularly important when the recommended agent is a new or infrequently employed drug.

Some drugs and medical devices presented in this publication have Food and Drug Administration (FDA) clearance for limited use in restricted research settings. It is the responsibility of the health care provider to ascertain the FDA status of each drug or device planned for use in their clinical practice.

To purchase additional copies of this book, call our customer service department at **(800) 638-3030** or fax orders to **(301) 223-2320**. International customers should call **(301) 223-2300**.

Visit Lippincott Williams & Wilkins on the Internet: http://www.lww.com. Lippincott Williams & Wilkins customer service representatives are available from 8:30 am to 6:00 pm, EST.

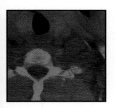

Introduction

Using the images from the corresponding text, this workbook allows students to work through a series of questions to evaluate their knowledge of sectional anatomy. In this second edition of *Introduction to Sectional Anatomy Workbook and Review Guide,* the cases have been expanded to include ultrasound images and updated to include the latest imaging technology including 3D and PET/CT. The organization of the patient images has been revised to enable the reader to more quickly compare images between the text and workbook. The images are numbered to correspond with the same image in the textbook.

Like the text, the workbook begins with an introductory chapter, followed by a chapter on the chest, since most students already have a basic knowledge and this chapter is relatively simple as compared to subsequent chapters. The chest is followed by the lower parts of the trunk, the abdomen, and pelvis. Once the students have become accustomed to learning sectional anatomy in the trunk, the more difficult regions of the body (head, neck, spine, and joints) are covered in the second half of the workbook.

To evaluate the students' knowledge, the series of multiple choice questions follow the format used on CT and MR registry examinations. After the extensive multiple choice questions, new Clinical Application questions have been added, including short answer and essay. Approximately eight case studies per chapter have also been added to give students samples of how their knowledge of sectional anatomy can be applied to patient exams, including CT, MR, PET/CT, and ultrasound (3D) images.

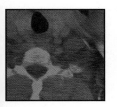

Contents

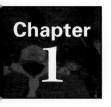

Introduction

LABELING EXERCISES

Fill in the blanks with the appropriate label.

A. The aortic arch demonstrating differences in axial sections taken at several levels (text Fig. 1-4).

B. The human body demonstrating planes of section (text Fig. 1-5).

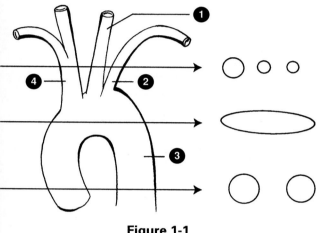

Figure 1-1

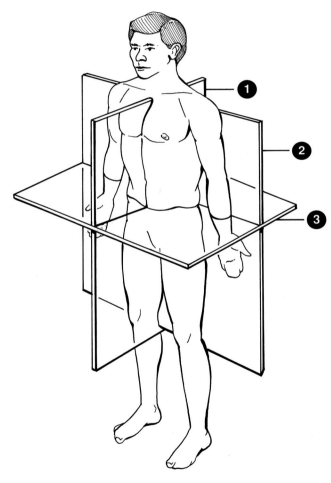

Figure 1-2

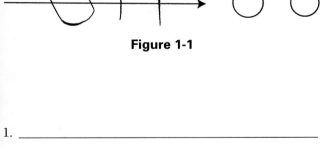

1. _____
2. _____
3. _____
4. _____

1. _____
2. _____
3. _____

C. Absorption values common to clinical radiology. The
   values shown are for the Electric and Musical
   Industries (EMI) and Hounsfield scales (text Fig. 1-6).

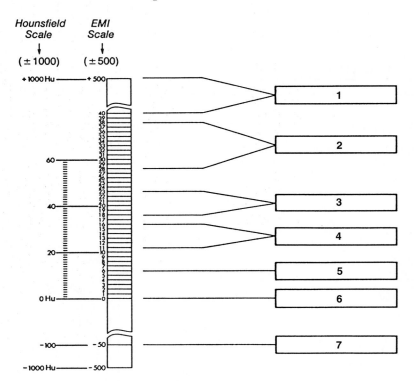

Figure 1-3

1. _____   5. _____

2. _____   6. _____

3. _____   7. _____

4. _____

CLINICAL APPLICATIONS

1. A plane or section dividing the body into upper and lower parts is classified as _____.

2. A plane or section dividing the body into equal right and left halves is classified as _____.

3. _____ is the classification of a hinge joint that allows movement in only one plane.

4. The hip and shoulder joints would be classified as _____.

5. Examples of the joint classification _____ include the sutures of the cranium and sternocostal joints.

6. Examples of the joint classification arthrodia include the _____ and _____ joints.

7. The wrist joint would be classified as _____.

8. Please list in order (from the most radiodense to the least radiodense) the following: fat, white matter, water, bone, and gray matter.

   _____

   _____

   _____

   _____

   _____

9. In a magnetic resonance (MR) image, a _____-weighted image will have a bright or high signal from water.

10. In a _____ scan, the metabolic activity and radiodensity of tissues are fused to create diagnostic images.

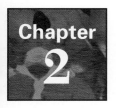

Chapter 2 Chest

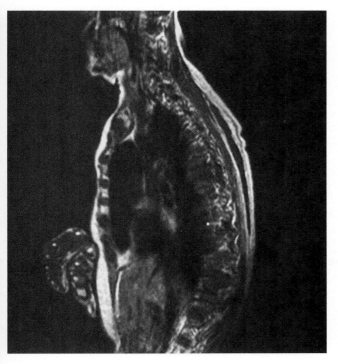
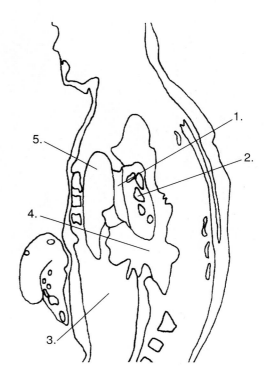

Figure 2-1

1. Which of the following is illustrated by 4?
   _____ A. Liver
   _____ B. Right lung lower lobe
   _____ C. Left lung lower lobe
   _____ D. Hilar region

2. Which of the following is illustrated by 2?
   _____ A. Aortic arch
   _____ B. Superior vena cava
   _____ C. Hilar region
   _____ D. Heart

3. What number illustrates the upper lobe of the lung?
   _____ A. 3
   _____ B. 1
   _____ C. 4
   _____ D. 5

4. Which of the following is illustrated by 3?
   _____ A. Stomach
   _____ B. Liver
   _____ C. Right lung lower lobe
   _____ D. Left lung lower lobe

5. What number illustrates the superior vena cava?
   _____ A. 1
   _____ B. 5
   _____ C. 4
   _____ D. 2

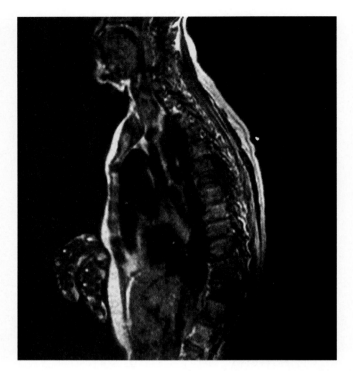

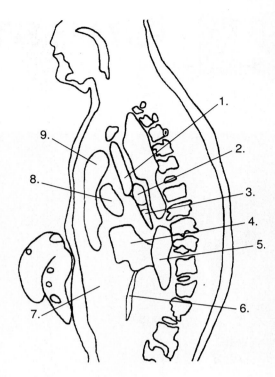

Figure 2-2

1. Which of the following is illustrated by 2?
   _____ A. Superior vena cava
   _____ B. Right pulmonary artery
   _____ C. Right pulmonary vein
   _____ D. Wall of the aortic arch

2. What number illustrates the inferior vena cava?
   _____ A. 5
   _____ B. 4
   _____ C. 3
   _____ D. 6

3. Which of the following is illustrated by 3?
   _____ A. Right pulmonary artery
   _____ B. Right pulmonary vein
   _____ C. Right atrium
   _____ D. Superior vena cava

4. What number illustrates the wall of the aortic arch?
   _____ A. 9
   _____ B. 7
   _____ C. 8
   _____ D. 1

5. Which of the following is illustrated by 4?
   _____ A. Liver
   _____ B. Right atrium
   _____ C. Right lung lower lobe
   _____ D. Inferior vena cava

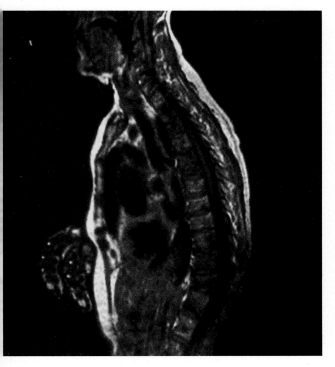 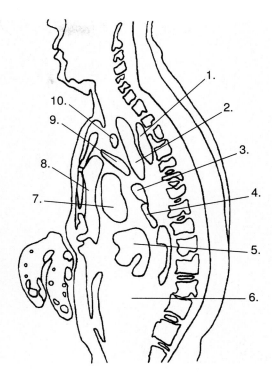

Figure 2-3

1. Which of the following is illustrated by 2?
   _____ A. Esophagus
   _____ B. Brachiocephalic artery
   _____ C. Trachea
   _____ D. Left brachiocephalic vein

2. What number illustrates the right lung upper lobe?
   _____ A. 7
   _____ B. 3
   _____ C. 8
   _____ D. 9

3. Which of the following is illustrated by 10?
   _____ A. Left brachiocephalic vein
   _____ B. Right brachiocephalic vein
   _____ C. Brachiocephalic artery
   _____ D. Left subclavian artery

4. Which of the following is illustrated by 4?
   _____ A. Right pulmonary artery
   _____ B. Left atrium
   _____ C. Right atrium
   _____ D. Left ventricle

5. What number illustrates the left brachiocephalic vein?
   _____ A. 10
   _____ B. 2
   _____ C. 9
   _____ D. 1

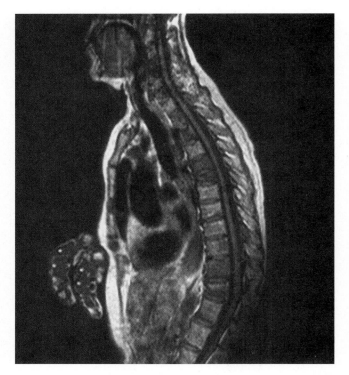 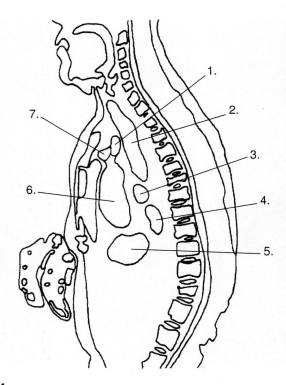

Figure 2-4

1. Which of the following is illustrated by 7?
   _____ A. Brachiocephalic artery
   _____ B. Left brachiocephalic vein
   _____ C. Aortic arch
   _____ D. Pulmonary artery

2. Which of the following is illustrated by 6?
   _____ A. Right pulmonary artery
   _____ B. Left atrium
   _____ C. Aortic arch
   _____ D. Left brachiocephalic vein

3. What number illustrates the brachiocephalic artery?
   _____ A. 1
   _____ B. 7
   _____ C. 3
   _____ D. 2

4. Which of the following is illustrated by 5?
   _____ A. Right pulmonary artery
   _____ B. Left atrium
   _____ C. Right atrium
   _____ D. Aortic arch

5. What number illustrates the right pulmonary artery?
   _____ A. 3
   _____ B. 6
   _____ C. 5
   _____ D. 4

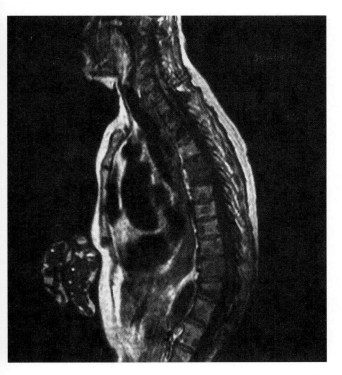
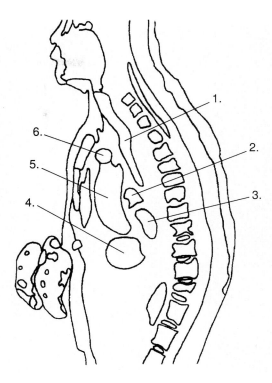

Figure 2-5

1. What number illustrates the right ventricle?
   _____ A. 6
   _____ B. 3
   _____ C. 4
   _____ D. 2

2. Which of the following is illustrated by 6?
   _____ A. Right pulmonary artery
   _____ B. Brachiocephalic artery
   _____ C. Aortic arch
   _____ D. Left brachiocephalic vein

3. Which of the following is illustrated by 5?
   _____ A. Left atrium
   _____ B. Right atrium
   _____ C. Aortic arch
   _____ D. Right ventricle

4. What number illustrates the right pulmonary artery?
   _____ A. 2
   _____ B. 6
   _____ C. 5
   _____ D. 3

5. Which of the following is illustrated by 3?
   _____ A. Right ventricle
   _____ B. Left atrium
   _____ C. Aortic arch
   _____ D. Right atrium

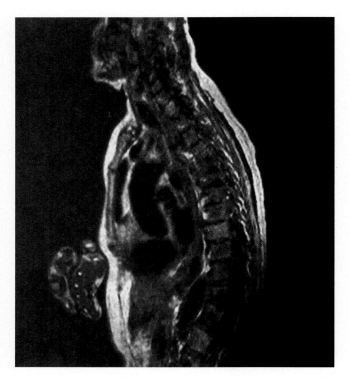 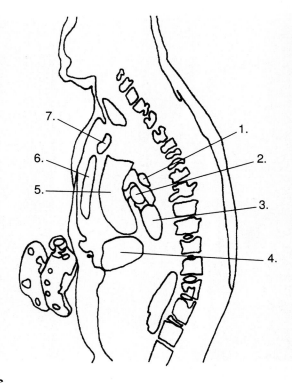

Figure 2-6

1. Which of the following is illustrated by 5?
   _____ A. Pleural cavity
   _____ B. Right atrium
   _____ C. Aortic arch
   _____ D. Left atrium

2. What number illustrates the left bronchus?
   _____ A. 1
   _____ B. 2
   _____ C. 5
   _____ D. 3

3. What number illustrates the pleural cavity?
   _____ A. 3
   _____ B. 4
   _____ C. 6
   _____ D. 5

4. Which of the following is illustrated by 2?
   _____ A. Left bronchus
   _____ B. Right pulmonary artery
   _____ C. Left atrium
   _____ D. Aortic arch

5. Which of the following is illustrated by 3?
   _____ A. Pleural cavity
   _____ B. Right ventricle
   _____ C. Left atrium
   _____ D. Aortic arch

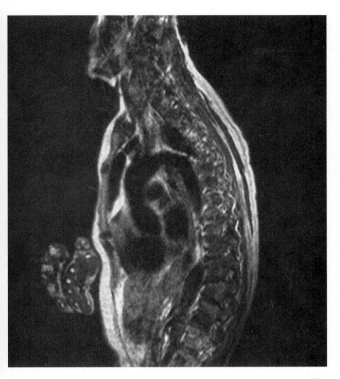
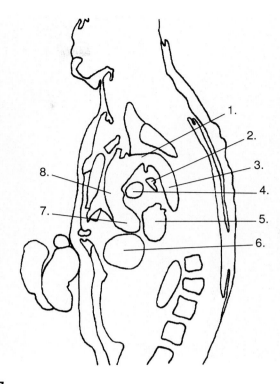

Figure 2-7

1. Which of the following is illustrated by 3?
   _____ A. Aortic arch
   _____ B. Left bronchus
   _____ C. Descending aorta
   _____ D. Pulmonary artery

2. What number illustrates the aortic arch?
   _____ A. 1
   _____ B. 4
   _____ C. 3
   _____ D. 2

3. Which of the following is illustrated by 7?
   _____ A. Left atrium
   _____ B. Right ventricle
   _____ C. Left ventricle
   _____ D. Ascending aorta

4. Which of the following is illustrated by 4?
   _____ A. Left bronchus
   _____ B. Descending aorta
   _____ C. Pulmonary artery
   _____ D. Left atrium

5. What number illustrates the ascending aorta?
   _____ A. 7
   _____ B. 5
   _____ C. 4
   _____ D. 8

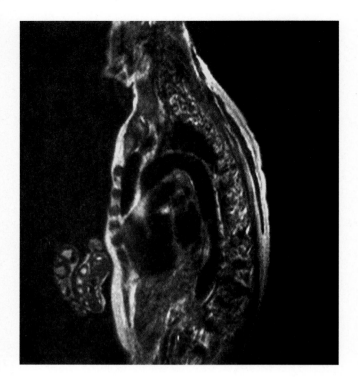

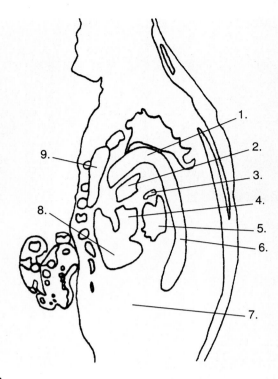

Figure 2-8

1. Which of the following is illustrated by 2?
   _____ A. Aortic arch
   _____ B. Pulmonary trunk
   _____ C. Right atrium
   _____ D. Left atrium

2. What number illustrates the right ventricle?
   _____ A. 2
   _____ B. 4
   _____ C. 8
   _____ D. 5

3. Which of the following is illustrated by 5?
   _____ A. Aortic arch
   _____ B. Left ventricle
   _____ C. Right ventricle
   _____ D. Left atrium

4. Which of the following is illustrated by 3?
   _____ A. Left bronchus
   _____ B. Left ventricle
   _____ C. Left atrium
   _____ D. Pulmonary trunk

5. What number illustrates the left ventricle?
   _____ A. 2
   _____ B. 5
   _____ C. 4
   _____ D. 8

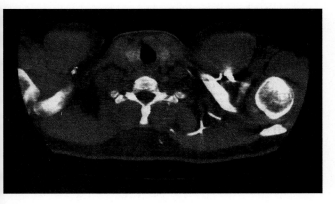 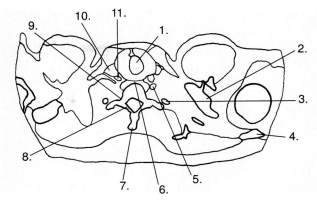

Figure 2-9

1. What number illustrates the right common carotid artery?
   _____ A. 10
   _____ B. 5
   _____ C. 3
   _____ D. 11

2. Which of the following is illustrated by 10?
   _____ A. Right external jugular vein
   _____ B. Right internal jugular vein
   _____ C. Right common carotid artery
   _____ D. Right subclavian artery

3. What number illustrates the clavicle?
   _____ A. 2
   _____ B. 4
   _____ C. 1
   _____ D. 8

4. Which of the following is illustrated by 9?
   _____ A. Spinous process of T1
   _____ B. Pedicle of T1
   _____ C. Transverse process of T1
   _____ D. Lamina of T1

5. Which of the following is illustrated by 6?
   _____ A. Thyroid
   _____ B. Trachea
   _____ C. Esophagus
   _____ D. Larynx

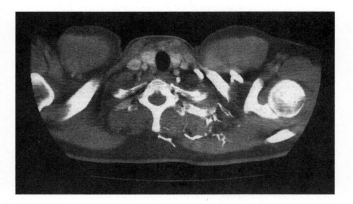
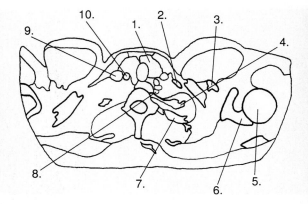

Figure 2-10

1. Which of the following is illustrated by 9?
   _____ A. Right internal jugular vein
   _____ B. Left subclavian vein
   _____ C. Left vertebral artery
   _____ D. Right common carotid artery

2. What number illustrates the first rib?
   _____ A. 6
   _____ B. 4
   _____ C. 7
   _____ D. 3

3. Which of the following is illustrated by 8?
   _____ A. Left subclavian vein
   _____ B. Left subclavian artery
   _____ C. Left vertebral artery
   _____ D. Left axillary vein

4. Which of the following is illustrated by 7?
   _____ A. Glenoid process of scapula
   _____ B. First rib
   _____ C. Second rib
   _____ D. Head of the humerus

5. What number illustrates the right common carotid artery?
   _____ A. 9
   _____ B. 8
   _____ C. 2
   _____ D. 10

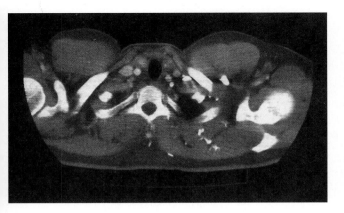 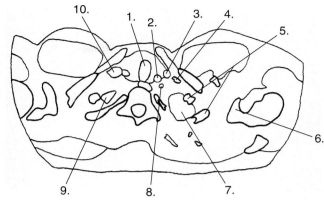

Figure 2-11

1. Which of the following is illustrated by 9?
   _____ A. Axillary vein
   _____ B. Upper lobe left lung
   _____ C. Upper lobe of right lung
   _____ D. Internal jugular vein

2. What number illustrates the coracoid process of the scapula?
   _____ A. 9
   _____ B. 6
   _____ C. 5
   _____ D. 1

3. What number illustrates the left vertebral artery?
   _____ A. 2
   _____ B. 8
   _____ C. 4
   _____ D. 3

4. Which of the following is illustrated by 4?
   _____ A. Left internal jugular vein
   _____ B. Left common carotid artery
   _____ C. Left axillary artery
   _____ D. Left subclavian vein

5. Which of the following is illustrated by 2?
   _____ A. Left common carotid artery
   _____ B. Trachea
   _____ C. Left subclavian vein
   _____ D. Left vertebral artery

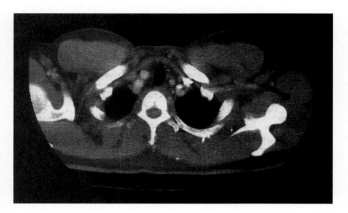 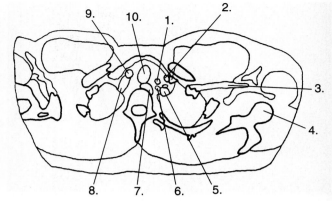

Figure 2-12

1. Which of the following is illustrated by 2?
   _____ A. Left common carotid artery
   _____ B. Left brachiocephalic vein
   _____ C. Left axillary artery
   _____ D. Left vertebral artery

2. What number illustrates the left axillary artery?
   _____ A. 3
   _____ B. 7
   _____ C. 6
   _____ D. 5

3. Which of the following is illustrated by 6?
   _____ A. Left subclavian artery
   _____ B. Left subclavian vein
   _____ C. Left vertebral artery
   _____ D. Left common carotid artery

4. What number illustrates the right common carotid artery?
   _____ A. 9
   _____ B. 10
   _____ C. 1
   _____ D. 8

5. Which of the following is illustrated by 1?
   _____ A. Left brachiocephalic vein
   _____ B. Left vertebral artery
   _____ C. Left subclavian artery
   _____ D. Left common carotid artery

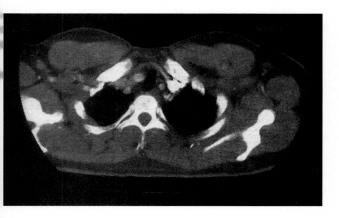 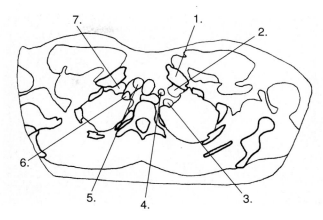

Figure 2-13

1. Which of the following is illustrated by 2?
   _____ A. Left clavicle
   _____ B. Left brachiocephalic vein
   _____ C. Left subclavian artery
   _____ D. Left common carotid artery

2. What number illustrates the origin of the right common carotid artery?
   _____ A. 7
   _____ B. 5
   _____ C. 6
   _____ D. 4

3. Which of the following is illustrated by 1?
   _____ A. Left clavicle
   _____ B. Left brachiocephalic vein
   _____ C. Left subclavian artery
   _____ D. Left common carotid artery

4. Which of the following is illustrated by 6?
   _____ A. Origin of the right vertebral artery
   _____ B. Origin of the right common carotid artery
   _____ C. Origin of the right subclavian artery
   _____ D. Right brachiocephalic vein

5. What number illustrates the left common carotid artery?
   _____ A. 2
   _____ B. 6
   _____ C. 4
   _____ D. 3

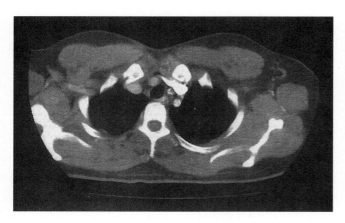 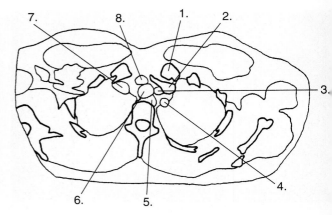

Figure 2-14

1. What number illustrates the brachiocephalic artery?
   _____ A. 7
   _____ B. 6
   _____ C. 4
   _____ D. 8

2. Which of the following is illustrated by 6?
   _____ A. Left subclavian artery
   _____ B. Esophagus
   _____ C. Trachea
   _____ D. Right brachiocephalic vein

3. Which of the following is illustrated by 4?
   _____ A. Left common carotid artery
   _____ B. Left subclavian artery
   _____ C. Left vertebral artery
   _____ D. Left axillary artery

4. What number illustrates the left brachiocephalic vein?
   _____ A. 2
   _____ B. 8
   _____ C. 1
   _____ D. 4

5. Which of the following is illustrated by 7?
   _____ A. Left brachiocephalic vein
   _____ B. Right subclavian vein
   _____ C. Brachiocephalic artery
   _____ D. Right brachiocephalic vein

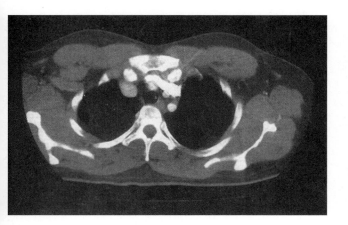 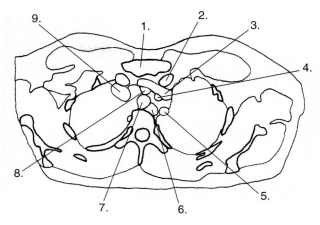

Figure 2-15

1. Which of the following is illustrated by 6?
   _____ A. Left subclavian artery
   _____ B. Esophagus
   _____ C. Trachea
   _____ D. Left common carotid artery

2. What number illustrates the right brachiocephalic vein?
   _____ A. 8
   _____ B. 7
   _____ C. 4
   _____ D. 9

3. Which of the following is illustrated by 1?
   _____ A. Clavicle
   _____ B. Trachea
   _____ C. Left brachiocephalic vein
   _____ D. Manubrium

4. Which of the following is illustrated by 4?
   _____ A. Left subclavian vein
   _____ B. Subclavian artery
   _____ C. Left common carotid artery
   _____ D. Left brachiocephalic vein

5. What number illustrates the brachiocephalic artery?
   _____ A. 9
   _____ B. 6
   _____ C. 8
   _____ D. 4

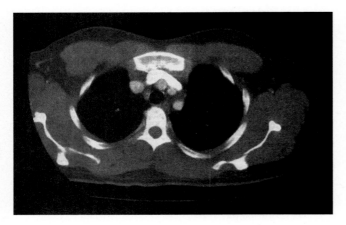
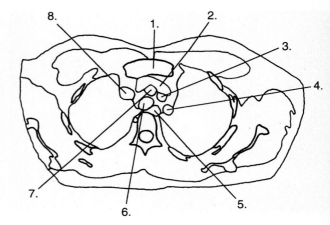

Figure 2-16

1. What number illustrates the left brachiocephalic vein?
_____ A. 2
_____ B. 8
_____ C. 7
_____ D. 4

2. Which of the following is illustrated by 5?
_____ A. Left common carotid artery
_____ B. Esophagus
_____ C. Trachea
_____ D. Manubrium

3. Which of the following is illustrated by 4?
_____ A. Left vertebral artery
_____ B. Brachiocephalic artery
_____ C. Left subclavian artery
_____ D. Left common carotid artery

4. What number illustrates the brachiocephalic artery?
_____ A. 4
_____ B. 2
_____ C. 3
_____ D. 7

5. Which of the following is illustrated by 6?
_____ A. Right brachiocephalic vein
_____ B. Esophagus
_____ C. Trachea
_____ D. Right internal jugular vein

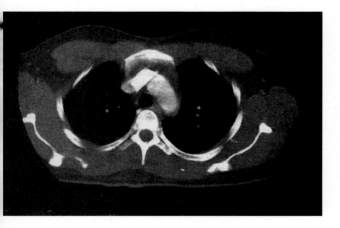 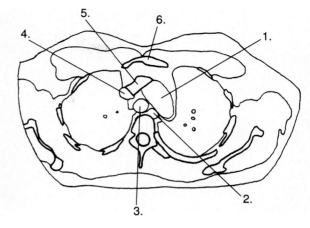

Figure 2-17

1. Which of the following is illustrated by 2?
   _____ A. Trachea
   _____ B. Vertebral artery
   _____ C. Aortic arch
   _____ D. Esophagus

2. What number illustrates the right brachiocephalic vein?
   _____ A. 5
   _____ B. 3
   _____ C. 4
   _____ D. 2

3. What number illustrates the aortic arch?
   _____ A. 1
   _____ B. 4
   _____ C. 5
   _____ D. 2

4. Which of the following is illustrated by 5?
   _____ A. Aortic arch
   _____ B. Left brachiocephalic vein
   _____ C. Brachiocephalic artery
   _____ D. Right brachiocephalic vein

5. Which of the following is illustrated by 3?
   _____ A. Aortic arch
   _____ B. Trachea
   _____ C. Esophagus
   _____ D. Left main bronchus

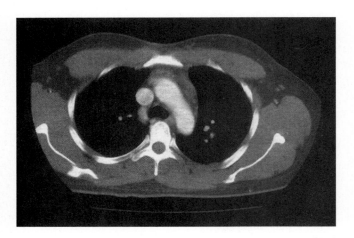 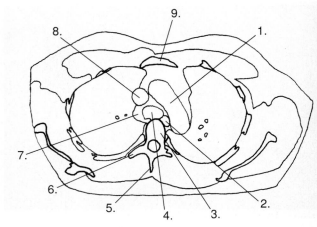

Figure 2-18

1. What number illustrates the azygos arch?
_____ A. 7
_____ B. 8
_____ C. 2
_____ D. 1

2. Which of the following is illustrated by 3?
_____ A. Esophagus
_____ B. Vertebral body
_____ C. Trachea
_____ D. Azygos arch

3. Which of the following is illustrated by 5?
_____ A. Pedicle
_____ B. Lamina
_____ C. Spinous process
_____ D. Transverse process

4. What number illustrates the transverse process?
_____ A. 7
_____ B. 5
_____ C. 6
_____ D. 1

5. Which of the following is illustrated by 8?
_____ A. Inferior vena cava
_____ B. Ascending aorta
_____ C. Azygos arch
_____ D. Superior vena cava

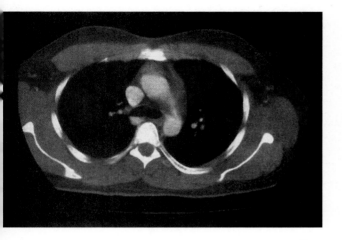 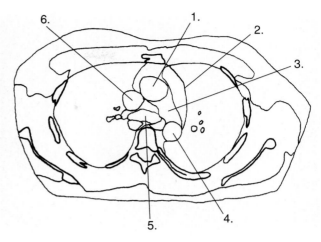

Figure 2-19

1. Which of the following is illustrated by 2?
   _____ A. Right atrium
   _____ B. Mediastinal pleura
   _____ C. Left atrium
   _____ D. Right ventricle

2. What number illustrates the tracheal bifurcation?
   _____ A. 6
   _____ B. 3
   _____ C. 5
   _____ D. 2

3. Which of the following is illustrated by 4?
   _____ A. Mediastinal pleura
   _____ B. Ascending aorta
   _____ C. Bottom of the aortic arch
   _____ D. Descending aorta

4. Which of the following is illustrated by l?
   _____ A. Ascending aorta
   _____ B. Bottom of the aortic arch
   _____ C. Superior vena cava
   _____ D. Descending aorta

5. What number illustrates the bottom of the aortic arch?
   _____ A. 5
   _____ B. 3
   _____ C. 4
   _____ D. 1

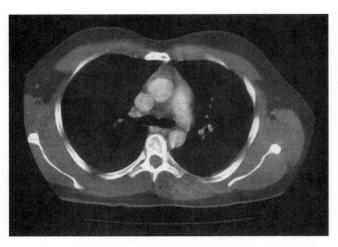 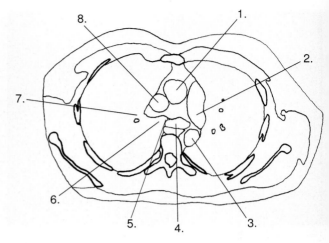

Figure 2-20

1. Which of the following is illustrated by 7?
   _____ A. Right main bronchus
   _____ B. Right lower lobe bronchus
   _____ C. Right upper lobe bronchus
   _____ D. Carina

2. What number illustrates the left main bronchus?
   _____ A. 7
   _____ B. 4
   _____ C. 5
   _____ D. 6

3. Which of the following is illustrated by 5?
   _____ A. Descending aorta
   _____ B. Carina
   _____ C. Left pulmonary artery
   _____ D. Ascending aorta

4. Which of the following is illustrated by 6?
   _____ A. Right main bronchus
   _____ B. Left main bronchus
   _____ C. Right lower lobe bronchus
   _____ D. Right upper lobe bronchus

5. What number illustrates the left pulmonary artery?
   _____ A. 8
   _____ B. 2
   _____ C. 3
   _____ D. 1

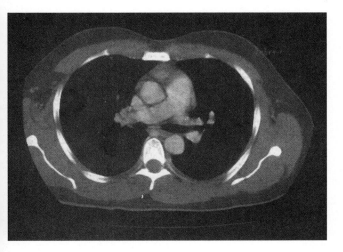 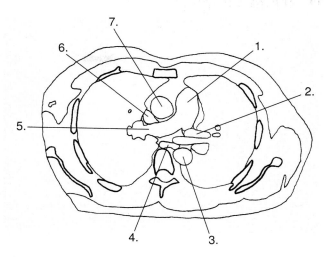

Figure 2-21

1. What number illustrates the esophagus?
   _____ A. 7
   _____ B. 4
   _____ C. 3
   _____ D. 2

2. Which of the following is illustrated by 5?
   _____ A. Pulmonary trunk
   _____ B. Left superior pulmonary vein
   _____ C. Ascending aorta
   _____ D. Right pulmonary artery

3. What number illustrates the left superior pulmonary vein?
   _____ A. 1
   _____ B. 2
   _____ C. 5
   _____ D. 3

4. Which of the following is illustrated by 1?
   _____ A. Left pulmonary artery
   _____ B. Ascending aorta
   _____ C. Pulmonary trunk
   _____ D. Descending aorta

5. Which of the following is illustrated by 6?
   _____ A. Ascending aorta
   _____ B. Left superior pulmonary vein
   _____ C. Descending aorta
   _____ D. Superior vena cava

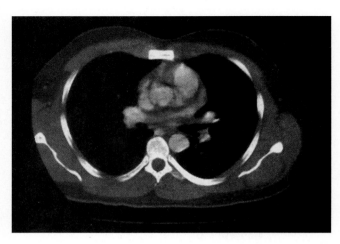 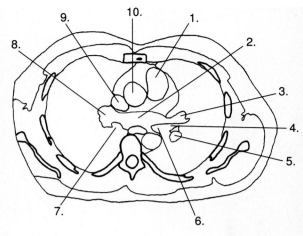

Figure 2-22

1. What number illustrates the left atrium?
   _____ A. 2
   _____ B. 9
   _____ C. 1
   _____ D. 10

2. Which of the following is illustrated by 7?
   _____ A. Left main bronchus
   _____ B. Bronchus intermedius
   _____ C. Superior pulmonary vein
   _____ D. Left upper lobe bronchus

3. What number illustrates the descending branch of the left pulmonary artery?
   _____ A. 6
   _____ B. 4
   _____ C. 5
   _____ D. 3

4. Which of the following is illustrated by 1?
   _____ A. Left superior pulmonary vein
   _____ B. Superior vena cava
   _____ C. Origin of the pulmonary trunk
   _____ D. Ascending aorta

5. Which of the following is illustrated by 4?
   _____ A. Left main bronchus
   _____ B. Descending branch of the left pulmonary artery
   _____ C. Left superior pulmonary vein
   _____ D. Left upper lobe bronchus

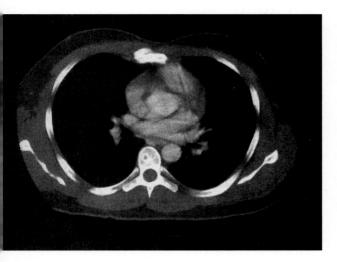 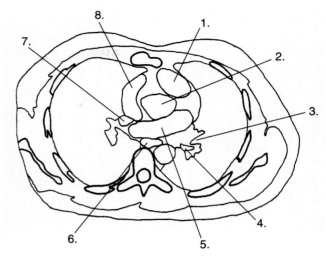

Figure 2-23

1. What number illustrates the ascending aorta?
   _____ A. 8
   _____ B. 2
   _____ C. 7
   _____ D. 1

2. Which of the following is illustrated by 4?
   _____ A. Left lower lobe bronchus
   _____ B. Left upper lobe bronchus
   _____ C. Left main bronchus
   _____ D. Carina

3. Which of the following is illustrated by 8?
   _____ A. Right ventricle
   _____ B. Right atrium
   _____ C. Right superior pulmonary vein
   _____ D. Left atrium

4. Which of the following is illustrated by 1?
   _____ A. Left atrium
   _____ B. Left ventricle
   _____ C. Right atrium
   _____ D. Right ventricle

5. What number illustrates the left atrium?
   _____ A. 8
   _____ B. 6
   _____ C. 5
   _____ D. 2

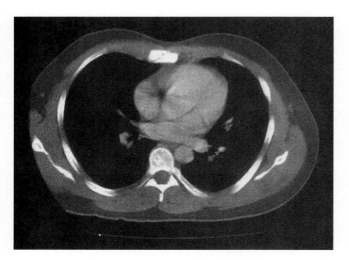

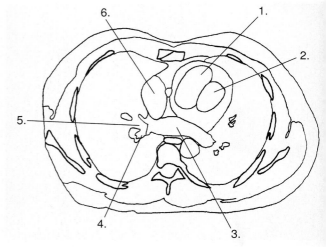

Figure 2-24

1. What number illustrates the left atrium?
   _____ A. 6
   _____ B. 2
   _____ C. 3
   _____ D. 1

2. Which of the following is illustrated by 4?
   _____ A. Right lower lobe bronchus
   _____ B. Right upper lobe bronchus
   _____ C. Right middle lobe bronchus
   _____ D. Carina

3. Which of the following is illustrated by 5?
   _____ A. Right upper lobe bronchus
   _____ B. Right lower lobe bronchus
   _____ C. Right middle lobe bronchus
   _____ D. Carina

4. What number illustrates the chamber within the heart responsible for pumping blood to the lungs?
   _____ A. 1
   _____ B. 6
   _____ C. 2
   _____ D. 3

5. Which of the following is illustrated by 6?
   _____ A. Left atrium
   _____ B. Right ventricle
   _____ C. Left ventricle
   _____ D. Right atrium

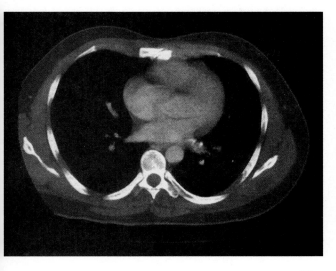
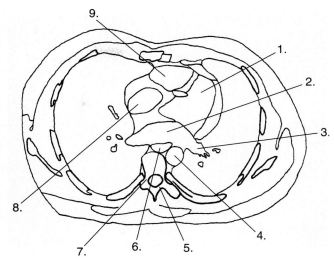

Figure 2-25

1. What number illustrates the lamina?
   _____ A. 7
   _____ B. 5
   _____ C. 6
   _____ D. 3

2. Which of the following is illustrated by 3?
   _____ A. Left atrium
   _____ B. Left inferior pulmonary vein
   _____ C. Left upper pulmonary vein
   _____ D. Hemiazygos vein

3. What number illustrates the right ventricle?
   _____ A. 8
   _____ B. 4
   _____ C. 1
   _____ D. 9

4. Which of the following is illustrated by 7?
   _____ A. Esophagus
   _____ B. Lamina
   _____ C. Pedicle
   _____ D. Descending aorta

5. Which of the following is illustrated by 1?
   _____ A. Left atrium
   _____ B. Right atrium
   _____ C. Left ventricle
   _____ D. Right ventricle

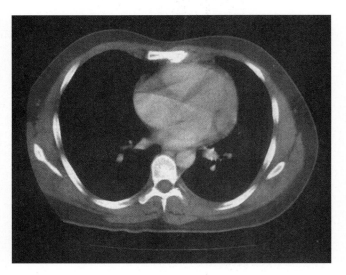
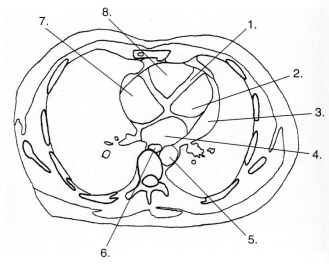

Figure 2-26

1. Which of the following is illustrated by 7?
   _____ A. Left atrium
   _____ B. Right atrium
   _____ C. Left ventricle
   _____ D. Right ventricle

2. Which of the following is illustrated by 8?
   _____ A. Right atrium
   _____ B. Left ventricle
   _____ C. Left atrium
   _____ D. Right ventricle

3. What number illustrates the descending aorta?
   _____ A. 4
   _____ B. 2
   _____ C. 5
   _____ D. 6

4. What number illustrates the ventricular wall?
   _____ A. 4
   _____ B. 3
   _____ C. 1
   _____ D. 6

5. Which of the following is illustrated by 4?
   _____ A. Left ventricle
   _____ B. Left atrium
   _____ C. Esophagus
   _____ D. Descending aorta

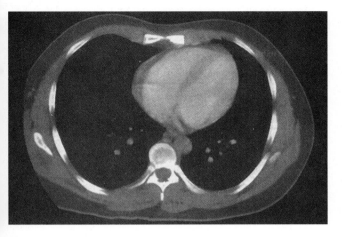
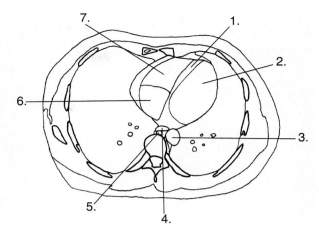

Figure 2-27

1. Which of the following is illustrated by 2?
   _____ A. Interventricular septum
   _____ B. Esophagus
   _____ C. Descending aorta
   _____ D. Left ventricle

2. What number illustrates the chamber of the heart receiving venous blood from the inferior vena cava?
   _____ A. 3
   _____ B. 2
   _____ C. 6
   _____ D. 7

3. Which of the following is illustrated by 5?
   _____ A. Accessory hemiazygos vein
   _____ B. Esophagus
   _____ C. Azygos vein
   _____ D. Hemiazygos vein

4. Which of the following is illustrated by 3?
   _____ A. Descending aorta
   _____ B. Hemiazygos vein
   _____ C. Azygos vein
   _____ D. Accessory hemiazygos vein

5. What number illustrates the right ventricle?
   _____ A. 2
   _____ B. 6
   _____ C. 3
   _____ D. 7

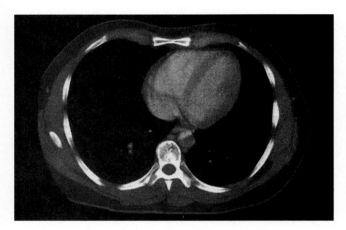 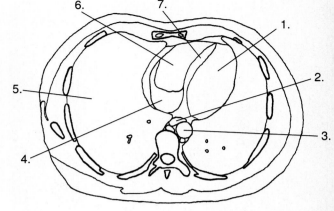

Figure 2-28

1. Which of the following is illustrated by 1?
   _____ A. Left atrium
   _____ B. Right ventricle
   _____ C. Left ventricle
   _____ D. Right atrium

2. Which of the following is illustrated by 5?
   _____ A. Left lung
   _____ B. Right lung
   _____ C. Right atrium
   _____ D. Right ventricle

3. What number illustrates the alimentary structure connecting the pharynx to the stomach?
   _____ A. 2
   _____ B. 3
   _____ C. 6
   _____ D. 4

4. What number illustrates the interventricular septum?
   _____ A. 2
   _____ B. 5
   _____ C. 4
   _____ D. 7

5. Which of the following is illustrated by 4?
   _____ A. Right atrium
   _____ B. Right ventricle
   _____ C. Left atrium
   _____ D. Left ventricle

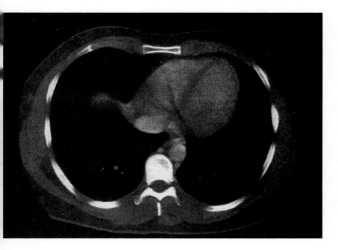 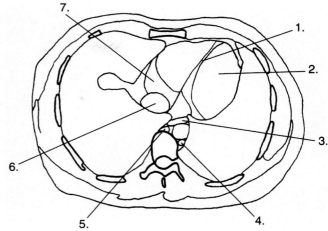

Figure 2-29

1. What number illustrates the inferior vena cava?
    _____ A. 3
    _____ B. 5
    _____ C. 4
    _____ D. 6

2. Which of the following is illustrated by 7?
    _____ A. Right ventricle
    _____ B. Right atrium
    _____ C. Inferior vena cava
    _____ D. Left ventricle

3. Which of the following is illustrated by 4?
    _____ A. Hemiazygos vein
    _____ B. Inferior vena cava
    _____ C. Azygos vein
    _____ D. Accessory hemiazygos vein

4. Which of the following is illustrated by 1?
    _____ A. Visceral peritoneum
    _____ B. Mediastinal pleura
    _____ C. Parietal peritoneum
    _____ D. Interventricular septum

5. What number illustrates the azygos vein?
    _____ A. 4
    _____ B. 3
    _____ C. 1
    _____ D. 5

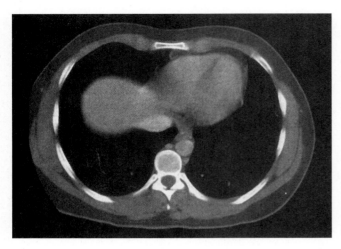

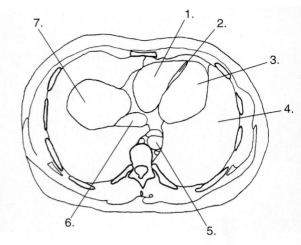

Figure 2-30

1. Which of the following is illustrated by 6?
   _____ A. Superior vena cava
   _____ B. Inferior vena cava
   _____ C. Right ventricle
   _____ D. Descending aorta

2. What number illustrates the interventricular septum?
   _____ A. 2
   _____ B. 6
   _____ C. 5
   _____ D. 4

3. What number illustrates the descending aorta?
   _____ A. 7
   _____ B. 3
   _____ C. 5
   _____ D. 6

4. Which of the following is illustrated by 7?
   _____ A. Left ventricle
   _____ B. Right ventricle
   _____ C. Stomach
   _____ D. Liver

5. Which of the following is illustrated by 3?
   _____ A. Left atrium
   _____ B. Left ventricle
   _____ C. Right ventricle
   _____ D. Liver

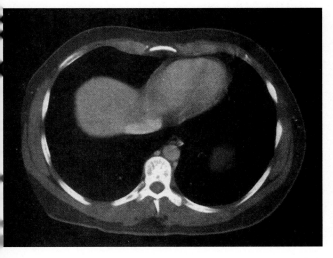 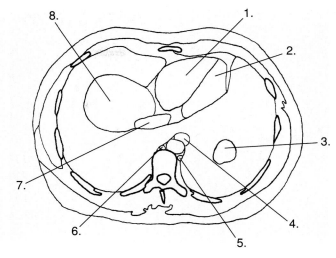

Figure 2-31

1. Which of the following is illustrated by 3?
   _____ A. Right ventricle
   _____ B. Left ventricle
   _____ C. Fundus of the stomach
   _____ D. Liver

2. What number illustrates the inferior vena cava?
   _____ A. 4
   _____ B. 6
   _____ C. 5
   _____ D. 7

3. Which of the following is illustrated by 6?
   _____ A. Azygos vein
   _____ B. Inferior vena cava
   _____ C. Hemiazygos vein
   _____ D. Accessory hemiazygos vein

4. What number illustrates the esophagus?
   _____ A. 3
   _____ B. 7
   _____ C. 6
   _____ D. 4

5. Which of the following is illustrated by 5?
   _____ A. Inferior vena cava
   _____ B. Accessory hemiazygos vein
   _____ C. Hemiazygos vein
   _____ D. Azygos vein

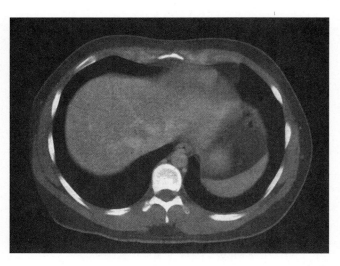

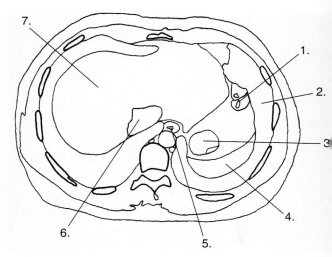

Figure 2-32

1. Which of the following is illustrated by 4?
   _____ A. Left lung
   _____ B. Spleen
   _____ C. Liver
   _____ D. Fundus of stomach

2. What number illustrates the vein transporting blood from the liver to the heart?
   _____ A. 5
   _____ B. 1
   _____ C. 3
   _____ D. 6

3. Which of the following is illustrated by 1?
   _____ A. Splenic flexure of the colon
   _____ B. Fundus of the stomach
   _____ C. Transverse colon
   _____ D. Spleen

4. Which of the following is illustrated by 3?
   _____ A. Spleen
   _____ B. Inferior vena cava
   _____ C. Esophagus
   _____ D. Fundus of the stomach

5. What number illustrates the left lung?
   _____ A. 2
   _____ B. 7
   _____ C. 6
   _____ D. 3

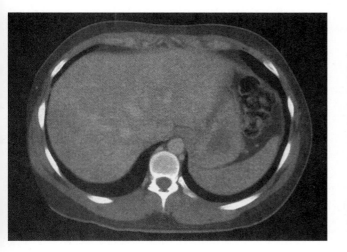 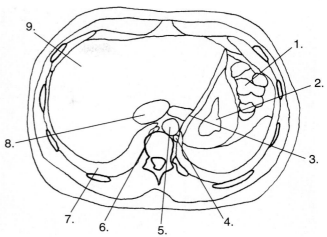

Figure 2-33

1. Which of the following is illustrated by 3?
   _____ A. Gastroesophageal junction
   _____ B. Spleen
   _____ C. Splenic flexure of colon
   _____ D. Liver

2. What number illustrates the splenic flexure of the colon?
   _____ A. 1
   _____ B. 8
   _____ C. 6
   _____ D. 3

3. Which of the following is illustrated by 6?
   _____ A. Accessory hemiazygos vein
   _____ B. Azygos vein
   _____ C. Hemiazygos vein
   _____ D. Inferior vena cava

4. Which of the following is illustrated by 5?
   _____ A. Esophagus
   _____ B. Inferior vena cava
   _____ C. Descending aorta
   _____ D. Azygos vein

5. What number illustrates the hemiazygos vein?
   _____ A. 5
   _____ B. 4
   _____ C. 8
   _____ D. 6

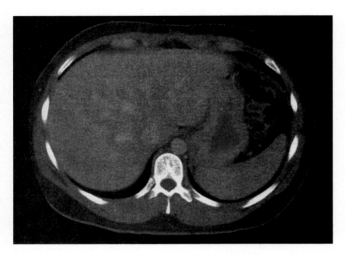

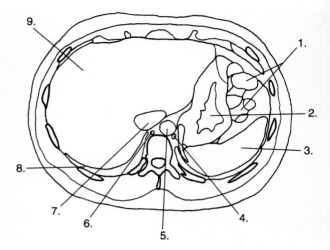

Figure 2-34

1. Which of the following is illustrated by 2?
   _____ A. Splenic flexure of colon
   _____ B. Fundus of stomach
   _____ C. Spleen
   _____ D. Body of stomach

2. What number illustrates the descending aorta?
   _____ A. 4
   _____ B. 2
   _____ C. 5
   _____ D. 6

3. Which of the following is illustrated by 3?
   _____ A. Spleen
   _____ B. Body of stomach
   _____ C. Liver
   _____ D. Splenic flexure of colon

4. Which of the following is illustrated by 7?
   _____ A. Spleen
   _____ B. Gallbladder
   _____ C. Descending aorta
   _____ D. Inferior vena cava

5. What number illustrates the splenic flexure of the colon?
   _____ A. 1
   _____ B. 5
   _____ C. 3
   _____ D. 2

CLINICAL APPLICATIONS

1. Which of the following does not originate from the aorta?
   _____ A. Brachiocephalic artery
   _____ B. Left subclavian artery
   _____ C. Left vertebral artery
   _____ D. Left common carotid artery

2. The pulmonary arteries carry deoxygenated blood. True or False?

3. The ascending aorta originates from what part of the heart?
   _____ A. Left ventricle
   _____ B. Left atrium
   _____ C. Right ventricle
   _____ D. Right atrium

4. Which of the following structures is located anterior to the hilum of the lungs?
   _____ A. Superior vena cava
   _____ B. Esophagus
   _____ C. Descending aorta
   _____ D. Accessory hemiazygos vein

5. The aorta arches over all of the following structures except the
   _____ A. Pulmonary trunk
   _____ B. Left brachiocephalic vein
   _____ C. Left main bronchus
   _____ D. Left pulmonary vein

6. In an axial section through the oblique fissure of the left lung, which lobe of the lung would be most anterior?

   _____

   _____

   _____

7. Which of the following structures is most posterior in the chest?
   _____ A. Trachea
   _____ B. Esophagus
   _____ C. Ascending aorta
   _____ D. Pulmonary trunk

8. Describe the left subclavian vein.

   _____

   _____

   _____

9. The vertebral arch consists of _____ pedicles, _____ laminae, and _____ processes (_____ transverse, _____ articular, and _____ spinous).

10. In a magnetic resonance (MR) image of the median sagittal chest, which chamber of the heart would be located most posteriorly?

    _____

    _____

    _____

CLINICAL CORRELATIONS

■ Clinical Case 2-1

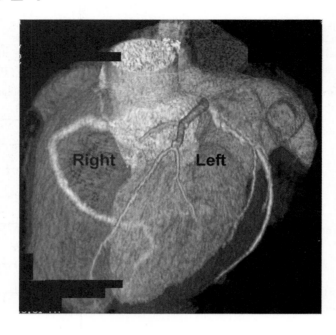

1. This image would best be described by which of the following:
   _____ A. Computed tomography angiography (CTA)
   _____ B. Magnetic resonance angiography (MRA)
   _____ C. Ultrasound
   _____ D. Positron emission tomography/computed tomography (PET/CT)

2. The anterior interventricular coronary artery originates from which of the following:
   _____ A. Right coronary artery
   _____ B. Left coronary artery

3. The right and left coronary arteries originate from which of the following:
   _____ A. Superior vena cava
   _____ B. Pulmonary veins
   _____ C. Pulmonary trunk
   _____ D. Ascending aorta

4. The _____ artery wraps around the heart to extend down the posterior side.
   _____ A. Anterior interventricular
   _____ B. Marginal
   _____ C. Circumflex
   _____ D. Posterior interventricular

5. The right coronary artery is found wrapping around the outside of the heart between the right atrium and

   _____ to reach the posterior side of the heart.
   _____ A. Right ventricle
   _____ B. Left atrium
   _____ C. Left ventricle
   _____ D. Aorta

■ Clinical Case 2-2

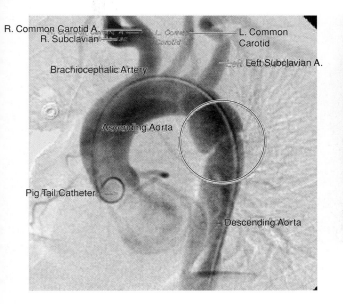

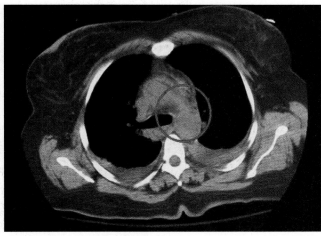

1. Describe the location of the false aneurysm resulting from trauma to the chest during a motor vehicle accident (MVA). The injury is shown with digital angiography (left) and axial CT (right) images.

   _____

   _____

   _____

2. Describe the changes in adjacent tissues.

   _____

   _____

   _____

3. Describe the consistency, shape, and border.

   _____

   _____

   _____

■ Clinical Case 2-3

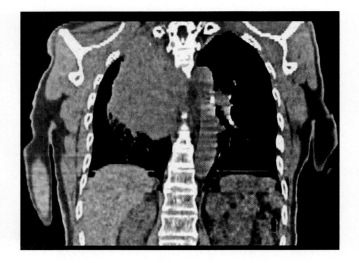

1. Describe the location of the non-small cell lung carcinoma (NSCLC) in this reconstructed coronal CT image.

   _____

   _____

   _____

2. Describe the changes in adjacent tissues.

   _____

   _____

   _____

3. Describe the consistency, shape, and border.

   _____

   _____

   _____

Clinical Case 2-4

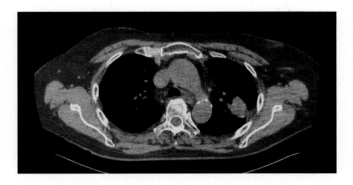

1. Describe the location of the primary pulmonary adeno-carcinoma in this selected axial CT image.

2. Describe the changes in adjacent tissues.

3. Describe the consistency, shape, and border.

■ Clinical Case 2-5

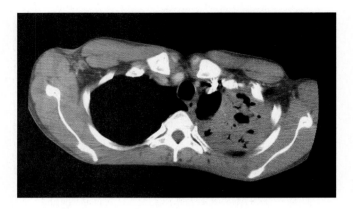

1. Describe the location of the necrotizing pneumonia as shown in this axial CT image.

   _____

   _____

   _____

2. Describe the changes in adjacent tissues.

   _____

   _____

   _____

3. Describe the consistency, shape, and border.

   _____

   _____

   _____

■ Clinical Case 2-6

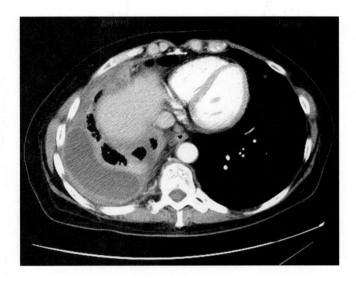

1. Describe the location of the pleural effusion found in this axial CT image.

   _____

   _____

   _____

2. Describe the changes in adjacent tissues.

   _____

   _____

   _____

3. Describe the consistency, shape, and border.

   _____

   _____

   _____

■ Clinical Case 2-7

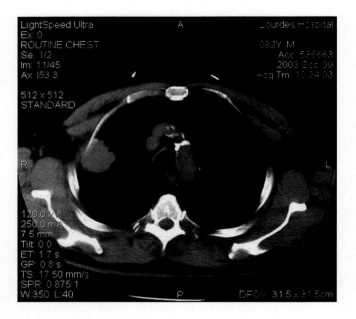

1. Describe the location of the malignant lung mass. Please note that the scan was done without contrast because the patient had a prior reaction to iodine.

   _____

   _____

   _____

2. Describe the changes in adjacent tissues.

   _____

   _____

   _____

3. Describe the consistency, shape, and border.

   _____

   _____

   _____

Abdomen

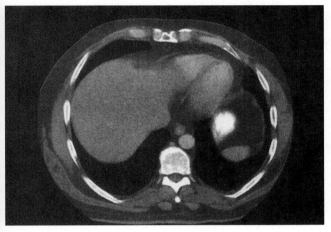

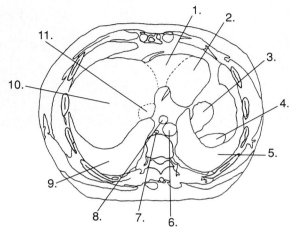

Figure 3-1

1. Which of the following is illustrated by 3?
   _____ A. Left ventricle
   _____ B. Inferior vena cava
   _____ C. Fundus of stomach
   _____ D. Spleen

2. Which of the following is illustrated by 10?
   _____ A. Left ventricle
   _____ B. Spleen
   _____ C. Right lung
   _____ D. Liver

3. What number illustrates the azygos vein?
   _____ A. 11
   _____ B. 6
   _____ C. 7
   _____ D. 3

4. What number illustrates the inferior vena cava?
   _____ A. 6
   _____ B. 8
   _____ C. 3
   _____ D. 11

5. Which of the following is illustrated by 4?
   _____ A. Spleen
   _____ B. Descending aorta
   _____ C. Esophagus
   _____ D. Inferior vena cava

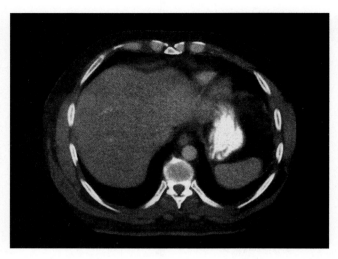

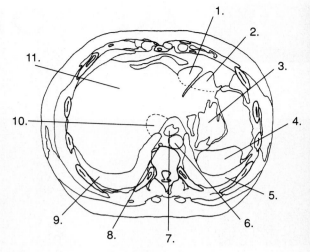

Figure 3-2

1. What number illustrates the chamber of the heart that pumps blood to most of the body?
   _____ A. 6
   _____ B. 2
   _____ C. 3
   _____ D. 1

2. Which of the following is illustrated by 5?
   _____ A. Right lung
   _____ B. Spleen
   _____ C. Left lung
   _____ D. Inferior vena cava

3. Which of the following is illustrated by 7?
   _____ A. Inferior vena cava
   _____ B. Esophagus
   _____ C. Descending aorta
   _____ D. Azygos vein

4. What number illustrates the liver?
   _____ A. 9
   _____ B. 4
   _____ C. 3
   _____ D. 11

5. Which of the following is illustrated by 1?
   _____ A. Quadrate lobe of liver
   _____ B. Right ventricle
   _____ C. Left ventricle
   _____ D. Gallbladder

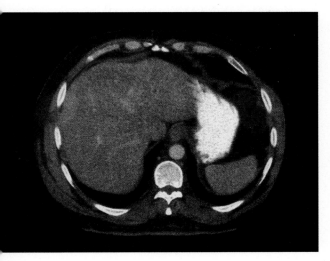 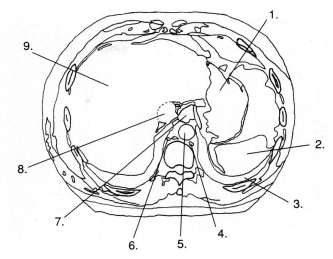

Figure 3-3

1. Which of the following is illustrated by 6?
   _____ A. Hemiazygos vein
   _____ B. Portal vein
   _____ C. Accessory hemiazygos vein
   _____ D. Azygos vein

2. Which of the following is illustrated by 1?
   _____ A. Spleen
   _____ B. Fundus of stomach
   _____ C. Quadrate lobe of liver
   _____ D. Esophagus

3. What number illustrates the hemiazygos vein?
   _____ A. 4
   _____ B. 7
   _____ C. 6
   _____ D. 5

4. Which of the following is illustrated by 8?
   _____ A. Descending aorta
   _____ B. Fundus of stomach
   _____ C. Inferior vena cava
   _____ D. Esophagus

5. What number illustrates the left lung?
   _____ A. 9
   _____ B. 2
   _____ C. 3
   _____ D. 1

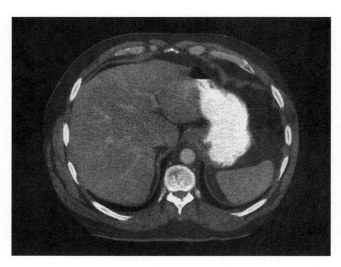 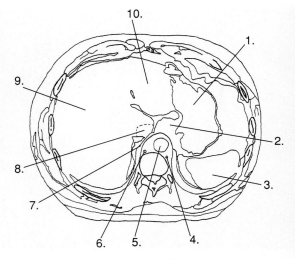

Figure 3-4

1. What number illustrates the body of the stomach?
   _____ A. 1
   _____ B. 9
   _____ C. 5
   _____ D. 2

2. Which of the following is illustrated by 7?
   _____ A. Hemiazygos vein
   _____ B. Right crus of diaphragm
   _____ C. Azygos vein
   _____ D. Right adrenal gland

3. What number illustrates the right lobe of the liver?
   _____ A. 10
   _____ B. 3
   _____ C. 9
   _____ D. 1

4. Which of the following is illustrated by 2?
   _____ A. Pancreas
   _____ B. Portal vein
   _____ C. Inferior vena cava
   _____ D. Gastroesophageal junction

5. Which of the following is illustrated by 6?
   _____ A. Hemiazygos vein
   _____ B. Azygos vein
   _____ C. Portal vein
   _____ D. Right crus of diaphragm

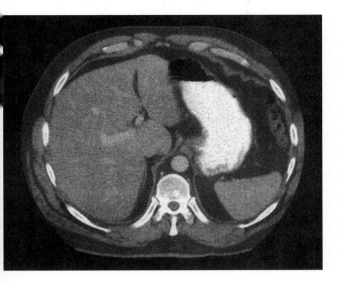

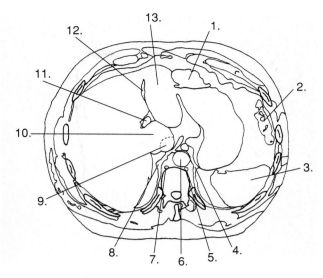

Figure 3-5

1. Which of the following is illustrated by 12?
   _____ A.   Quadrate lobe of liver
   _____ B.   Caudate lobe of liver
   _____ C.   Inferior vena cava
   _____ D.   Ligamentum teres fossa

2. What number illustrates the caudate lobe of liver?
   _____ A.   13
   _____ B.   3
   _____ C.   10
   _____ D.   1

3. Which of the following is illustrated by 2?
   _____ A.   Air in stomach
   _____ B.   Transverse colon
   _____ C.   Ascending colon
   _____ D.   Splenic flexure of colon

4. Which of the following is illustrated by 6?
   _____ A.   Descending aorta
   _____ B.   Celiac trunk
   _____ C.   Inferior vena cava
   _____ D.   Portal vein

5. What number illustrates the left lobe of liver?
   _____ A.   1
   _____ B.   10
   _____ C.   6
   _____ D.   13

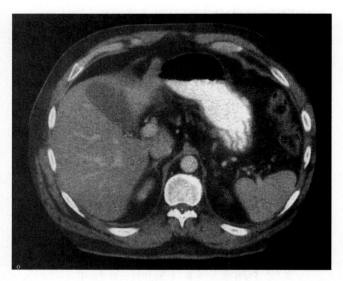
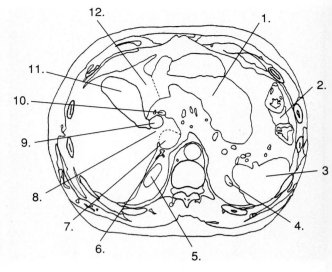

Figure 3-6

1. Which of the following is illustrated by 4?
   _____ A. Splenic vein
   _____ B. Upper pole of left kidney
   _____ C. Left adrenal gland
   _____ D. Inferior mesenteric vein

2. What number illustrates the adrenal gland?
   _____ A. 6
   _____ B. 9
   _____ C. 7
   _____ D. 5

3. What number illustrates the gallbladder?
   _____ A. 7
   _____ B. 9
   _____ C. 12
   _____ D. 11

4. Which of the following is illustrated by 12?
   _____ A. Left lobe of liver
   _____ B. Caudate lobe of liver
   _____ C. Gallbladder
   _____ D. Quadrate lobe of liver

5. Which of the following is illustrated by 10?
   _____ A. Common hepatic artery
   _____ B. Proper hepatic artery
   _____ C. Portal vein
   _____ D. Gastroduodenal artery

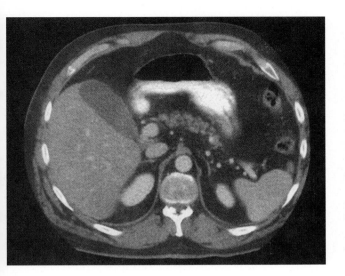
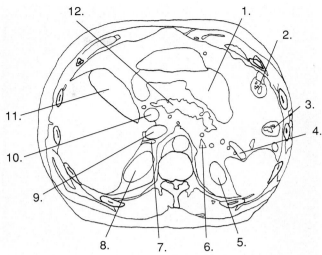

Figure 3-7

1. What number illustrates the descending colon?
   _____ A. 9
   _____ B. 3
   _____ C. 1
   _____ D. 2

2. Which of the following is illustrated by 7?
   _____ A. Upper pole of right kidney
   _____ B. Inferior vena cava
   _____ C. Splenic vein
   _____ D. Right adrenal gland

3. Which of the following is illustrated by 10?
   _____ A. Transverse colon
   _____ B. Inferior vena cava
   _____ C. Portal vein
   _____ D. Proper hepatic artery

4. Which of the following is illustrated by 2?
   _____ A. Descending colon
   _____ B. Splenic vein
   _____ C. Transverse colon
   _____ D. Left adrenal

5. What number illustrates the body of the pancreas?
   _____ A. 11
   _____ B. 1
   _____ C. 8
   _____ D. 12

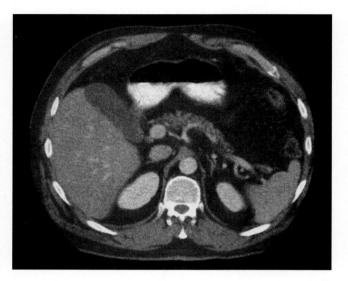

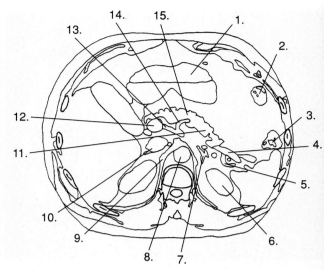

Figure 3-8

1. Which of the following is illustrated by 13?
　　_____ A. Hepatic artery
　　_____ B. Splenic artery
　　_____ C. Celiac trunk
　　_____ D. Cystic duct

2. What number illustrates the transverse colon?
　　_____ A. 2
　　_____ B. 3
　　_____ C. 1
　　_____ D. 15

3. Which of the following is illustrated by 11?
　　_____ A. Body of pancreas
　　_____ B. Stomach
　　_____ C. Duodenum
　　_____ D. Tail of pancreas

4. Which of the following is illustrated by 6?
　　_____ A. Left adrenal gland
　　_____ B. Left kidney
　　_____ C. Splenic flexure of colon
　　_____ D. Spleen

5. What number illustrates the splenic artery?
　　_____ A. 13
　　_____ B. 5
　　_____ C. 4
　　_____ D. 7

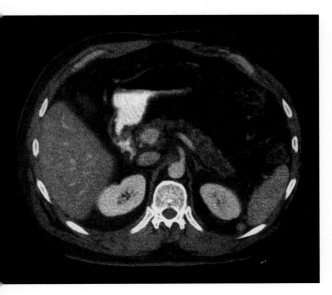
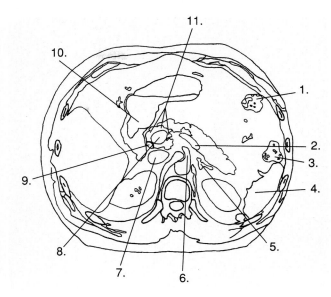

Figure 3-9

1. Which of the following is illustrated by 9?
   _____ A. Superior mesenteric artery
   _____ B. Hepatic artery
   _____ C. Portal vein
   _____ D. Common bile duct

2. What number illustrates the celiac trunk?
   _____ A. 8
   _____ B. 6
   _____ C. 5
   _____ D. 7

3. Which of the following is illustrated by 4?
   _____ A. Left adrenal gland
   _____ B. Inferior vena cava
   _____ C. Spleen
   _____ D. Head of pancreas

4. What number illustrates the pyloric antrum of the stomach?
   _____ A. 6
   _____ B. 1
   _____ C. 3
   _____ D. 10

5. Which of the following is illustrated by 11?
   _____ A. Head of pancreas
   _____ B. Pyloric antrum of stomach
   _____ C. Common bile duct
   _____ D. Duodenum

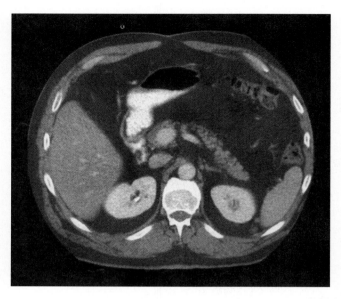

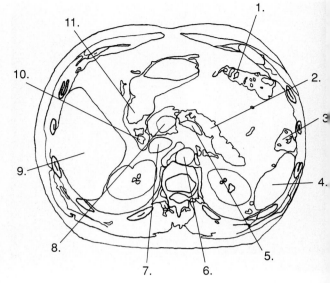

Figure 3-10

1. Which of the following is illustrated by 2?
   _____ A. Splenic vein
   _____ B. Body of pancreas
   _____ C. Portal vein
   _____ D. Duodenum

2. What number illustrates the first part of the small bowel?
   _____ A. 7
   _____ B. 2
   _____ C. 11
   _____ D. 10

3. What number illustrates the descending or abdominal aorta?
   _____ A. 7
   _____ B. 2
   _____ C. 6
   _____ D. 5

4. Which of the following is illustrated by 9?
   _____ A. Liver
   _____ B. Spleen
   _____ C. Body of pancreas
   _____ D. Pyloric antrum of stomach

5. Which of the following is illustrated by 1?
   _____ A. Descending colon
   _____ B. Transverse colon
   _____ C. Ascending colon
   _____ D. Duodenum

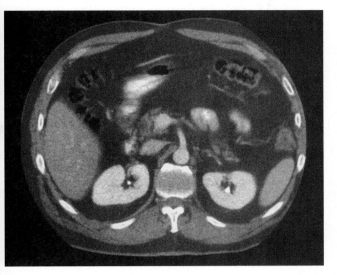 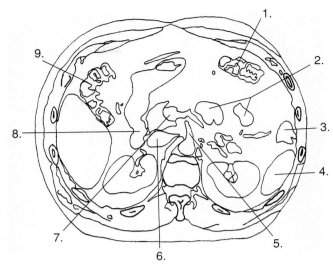

Figure 3-11

1. What number illustrates the vein carrying nutrient-rich venous blood to the liver?
   _____ A. 6
   _____ B. 5
   _____ C. 8
   _____ D. 7

2. Which of the following is illustrated by 9?
   _____ A. Transverse colon
   _____ B. Duodenum
   _____ C. Hepatic flexure at colon
   _____ D. Descending colon

3. Which of the following is illustrated by 5?
   _____ A. Celiac trunk
   _____ B. Superior mesenteric artery
   _____ C. Inferior mesenteric artery
   _____ D. Inferior vena cava

4. What number illustrates the descending colon?
   _____ A. 3
   _____ B. 1
   _____ C. 9
   _____ D. 4

5. Which of the following is illustrated by 4?
   _____ A. Adrenal gland
   _____ B. Ascending colon
   _____ C. Spleen
   _____ D. Liver

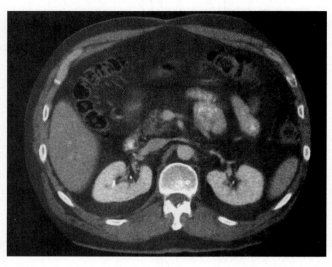
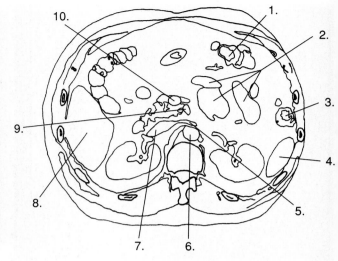

Figure 3-12

1. Which of the following is illustrated by 10?
   _____ A. Portal vein
   _____ B. Common bile duct
   _____ C. Superior mesenteric artery
   _____ D. Superior mesenteric vein

2. Which of the following is illustrated by 5?
   _____ A. Inferior mesenteric vein
   _____ B. Left renal vein
   _____ C. Crus of diaphragm
   _____ D. Superior mesenteric vein

3. What number illustrates the loops of the small bowel?
   _____ A. 3
   _____ B. 2
   _____ C. 4
   _____ D. 1

4. What number illustrates the superior mesenteric artery?
   _____ A. 10
   _____ B. 5
   _____ C. 9
   _____ D. 7

5. Which of the following is illustrated by 3?
   _____ A. Loops of small bowel
   _____ B. Ascending colon
   _____ C. Transverse colon
   _____ D. Descending colon

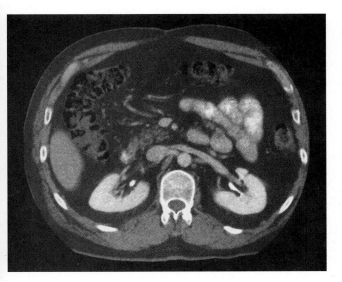

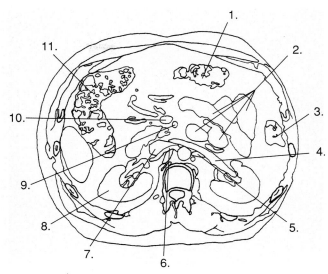

Figure 3-13

1. Which of the following is illustrated by 4?
   _____ A. Left renal vein
   _____ B. Renal artery
   _____ C. Inferior mesenteric vein
   _____ D. Inferior mesenteric artery

2. What number illustrates the inferior vena cava?
   _____ A. 6
   _____ B. 9
   _____ C. 7
   _____ D. 5

3. Which of the following is illustrated by 8?
   _____ A. Adrenal gland
   _____ B. Kidney
   _____ C. Loops of small bowel
   _____ D. Hepatic flexure of colon

4. What number illustrates the hepatic flexure of the colon?
   _____ A. 3
   _____ B. 8
   _____ C. 1
   _____ D. 11

5. Which of the following is illustrated by 5?
   _____ A. Renal vein
   _____ B. Renal artery
   _____ C. Superior mesenteric vein
   _____ D. Superior mesenteric artery

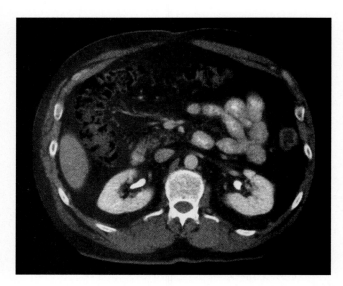
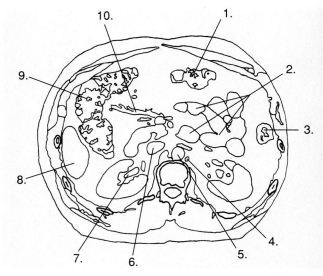

Figure 3-14

1. Which of the following is illustrated by 8?
   _____ A. Descending colon
   _____ B. Spleen
   _____ C. Liver
   _____ D. Adrenal gland

2. What number illustrates the hemiazygos vein?
   _____ A. 4
   _____ B. 5
   _____ C. 7
   _____ D. 6

3. What number illustrates the right renal pelvis?
   _____ A. 8
   _____ B. 6
   _____ C. 7
   _____ D. 5

4. Which of the following is illustrated by 10?
   _____ A. Portal vein
   _____ B. Loops of small bowel
   _____ C. Common bile duct
   _____ D. Mesenteric vessels

5. Which of the following is illustrated by 5?
   _____ A. Hemiazygos vein
   _____ B. Descending aorta
   _____ C. Inferior vena cava
   _____ D. Inferior mesenteric artery

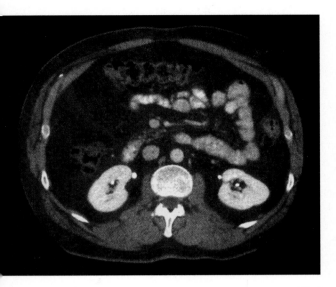
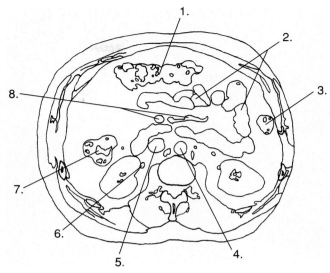

Figure 3-15

1. What number illustrates the abdominal aorta?
   _____ A. 4
   _____ B. 8
   _____ C. 5
   _____ D. 6

2. Which of the following is illustrated by 6?
   _____ A. Right renal vein
   _____ B. Right renal artery
   _____ C. Right ureter
   _____ D. Azygos vein

3. Which of the following is illustrated by 8?
   _____ A. Celiac vessels
   _____ B. Superior mesenteric vessels
   _____ C. Inferior mesenteric vessels
   _____ D. Loops of small bowel

4. Which of the following is illustrated by 3?
   _____ A. Ascending colon
   _____ B. Small bowel
   _____ C. Cecum
   _____ D. Descending colon

5. What number illustrates the ascending colon?
   _____ A. 2
   _____ B. 1
   _____ C. 3
   _____ D. 7

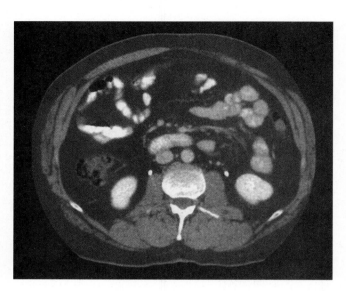 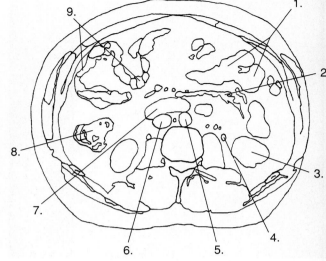

Figure 3-16

1. Which of the following is illustrated by 1?
   _____ A. Ascending colon
   _____ B. Transverse colon
   _____ C. Descending colon
   _____ D. Loops of small bowel

2. Which of the following is illustrated by 3?
   _____ A. Adrenal gland
   _____ B. Lower pole of left kidney
   _____ C. Ascending colon
   _____ D. Spleen

3. What number illustrates the duodenum?
   _____ A. 3
   _____ B. 1
   _____ C. 6
   _____ D. 7

4. What number illustrates the inferior vena cava?
   _____ A. 5
   _____ B. 4
   _____ C. 6
   _____ D. 7

5. Which of the following is illustrated by 4?
   _____ A. Left ureter
   _____ B. Left renal vein
   _____ C. Left renal artery
   _____ D. Hemiazygos vein

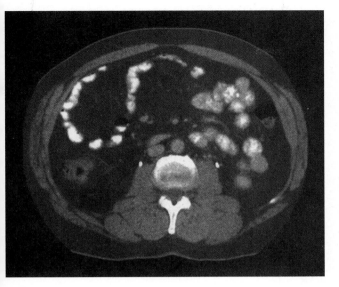
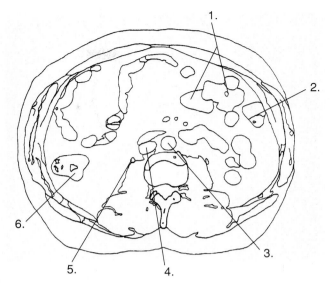

Figure 3-17

1. What number illustrates the abdominal aorta?
   _____ A. 3
   _____ B. 6
   _____ C. 5
   _____ D. 4

2. Which of the following is illustrated by 6?
   _____ A. Small bowel
   _____ B. Ascending colon
   _____ C. Descending colon
   _____ D. Cecum

3. What number illustrates the inferior vena cava?
   _____ A. 5
   _____ B. 2
   _____ C. 4
   _____ D. 3

4. Which of the following is illustrated by 2?
   _____ A. Loops of small bowel
   _____ B. Ascending colon
   _____ C. Cecum
   _____ D. Descending colon

5. Which of the following is illustrated by 5?
   _____ A. Inferior mesenteric artery
   _____ B. Right ureter
   _____ C. Interior mesenteric vein
   _____ D. Right renal artery

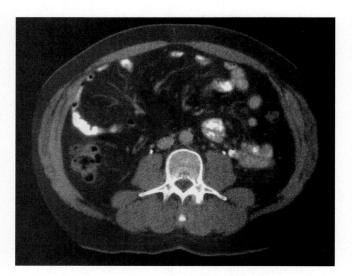

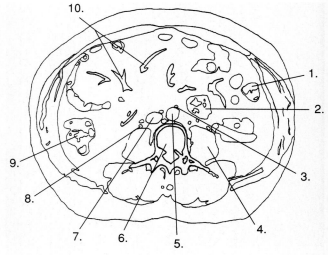

Figure 3-18

1. Which of the following is illustrated by 3?
   _____ A. Superior mesenteric artery
   _____ B. Inferior mesenteric artery
   _____ C. Celiac trunk
   _____ D. Ureter

2. Which of the following is illustrated by 1?
   _____ A. Ascending colon
   _____ B. Small bowel
   _____ C. Descending colon
   _____ D. Cecum

3. What number illustrates the ascending colon?
   _____ A. 10
   _____ B. 1
   _____ C. 2
   _____ D. 9

4. Which of the following is illustrated by 2?
   _____ A. Small bowel
   _____ B. Descending colon
   _____ C. Transverse colon
   _____ D. Ascending colon

5. What number illustrates the inferior mesenteric artery?
   _____ A. 7
   _____ B. 10
   _____ C. 8
   _____ D. 3

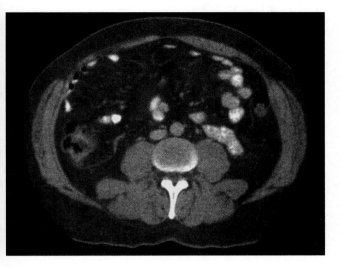 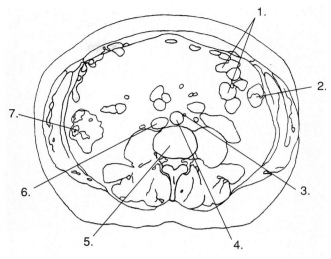

Figure 3-19

1. What number illustrates the loops of the small bowel?
   _____ A. 1
   _____ B. 7
   _____ C. 2
   _____ D. 4

2. Which of the following is illustrated by 5?
   _____ A. Psoas muscle
   _____ B. Vertebral body of L3
   _____ C. Intervertebral disk
   _____ D. Vertebral body of L4

3. Which of the following is illustrated by 7?
   _____ A. Descending colon
   _____ B. Ascending colon
   _____ C. Small bowel
   _____ D. Cecum

4. What number illustrates the abdominal aorta?
   _____ A. 2
   _____ B. 1
   _____ C. 4
   _____ D. 6

5. Which of the following is illustrated by 2?
   _____ A. Descending colon
   _____ B. Small bowel
   _____ C. Ascending colon
   _____ D. Cecum

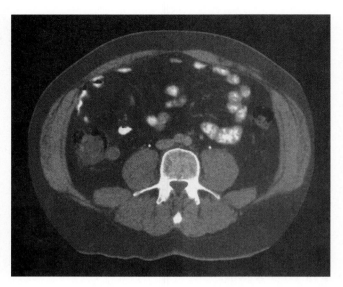 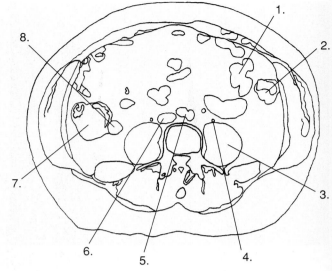

Figure 3-20

1. Which of the following is illustrated by 3?
   _____ A. Iliacus muscle
   _____ B. Psoas muscle
   _____ C. Ascending colon
   _____ D. Cecum

2. What number illustrates the common iliac arteries?
   _____ A. 6
   _____ B. 2
   _____ C. 5
   _____ D. 4

3. Which of the following is illustrated by 8?
   _____ A. Cecum
   _____ B. Descending colon
   _____ C. Ileum
   _____ D. Jejunum

4. Which of the following is illustrated by 7?
   _____ A. Descending colon
   _____ B. Ascending colon
   _____ C. Small bowel
   _____ D. Cecum

5. What number illustrates the small bowel?
   _____ A. 1
   _____ B. 3
   _____ C. 2
   _____ D. 7

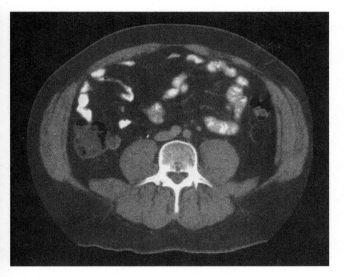

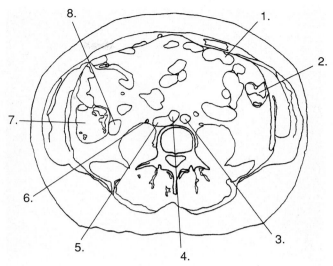

Figure 3-21

1. What number illustrates the ureter?
   _____ A. 4
   _____ B. 3
   _____ C. 5
   _____ D. 6

2. Which of the following is illustrated by 8?
   _____ A. Right common iliac artery
   _____ B. Cecum
   _____ C. Ileum
   _____ D. Jejunum

3. Which of the following is illustrated by 4?
   _____ A. Inferior mesenteric artery
   _____ B. Right common iliac artery
   _____ C. Inferior mesenteric vein
   _____ D. Inferior vena cava

4. Which of the following is illustrated by 2?
   _____ A. Small bowel
   _____ B. Descending colon
   _____ C. Ascending colon
   _____ D. Cecum

5. What number illustrates the left common iliac artery?
   _____ A. 3
   _____ B. 8
   _____ C. 4
   _____ D. 5

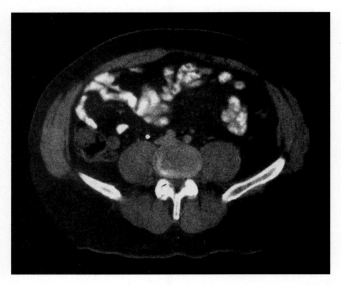 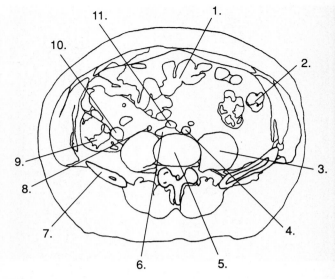

Figure 3-22

1. Which of the following is illustrated by 8?
   _____ A. Left common iliac artery
   _____ B. Ureter
   _____ C. Inferior mesenteric artery
   _____ D. Right common iliac artery

2. What number illustrates the psoas muscle?
   _____ A. 3
   _____ B. 10
   _____ C. 7
   _____ D. 5

3. What number illustrates the iliac crest?
   _____ A. 9
   _____ B. 1
   _____ C. 7
   _____ D. 4

4. Which of the following is illustrated by 5?
   _____ A. Vertebral body of L3
   _____ B. Intervertebral disk
   _____ C. Vertebral body of L4
   _____ D. Sacrum

5. Which of the following is illustrated by 6?
   _____ A. Left common iliac artery
   _____ B. Right common iliac artery
   _____ C. Inferior mesenteric vein
   _____ D. Inferior vena cava

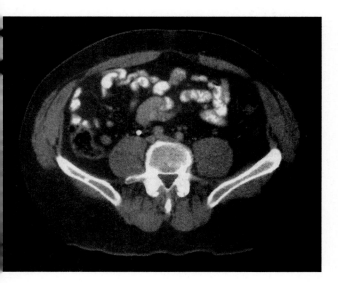 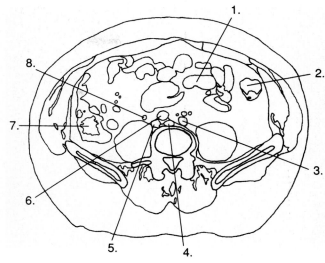

Figure 3-23

1. What number illustrates the small bowel?
_____ A. 1
_____ B. 6
_____ C. 2
_____ D. 7

2. Which of the following is illustrated by 4?
_____ A. Left common iliac artery
_____ B. Right common iliac vein
_____ C. Left common iliac vein
_____ D. Right common iliac artery

3. What number illustrates the right common iliac vein?
_____ A. 6
_____ B. 4
_____ C. 5
_____ D. 3

4. Which of the following is illustrated by 8?
_____ A. Right common iliac vein
_____ B. Right common iliac artery
_____ C. Right ureter
_____ D. Inferior mesenteric vein

5. Which of the following is illustrated by 2?
_____ A. Cecum
_____ B. Ascending colon
_____ C. Loops of small bowel
_____ D. Descending colon

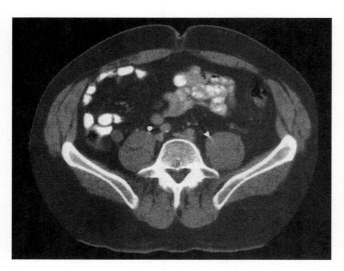
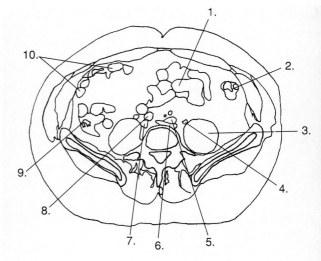

Figure 3-24

1. Which of the following is illustrated by 3?
   _____ A. Small bowel
   _____ B. Psoas muscle
   _____ C. Right common iliac vein
   _____ D. Cecum

2. What number illustrates the cecum?
   _____ A. 2
   _____ B. 3
   _____ C. 1
   _____ D. 9

3. What number illustrates the ureter?
   _____ A. 4
   _____ B. 8
   _____ C. 7
   _____ D. 5

4. Which of the following is illustrated by 1?
   _____ A. Cecum
   _____ B. Left psoas muscle
   _____ C. Small bowel
   _____ D. Transverse colon

5. Which of the following is illustrated by 7?
   _____ A. Ureter
   _____ B. Right common iliac vein
   _____ C. Right internal iliac vein
   _____ D. Right common iliac artery

CLINICAL APPLICATIONS

1. The boundary of the upper abdomen is formed by the _____, and the lower abdomen extends into the_____.

2. Which of the following is located most superiorly?
   _____ A. Transverse colon
   _____ B. Hepatic flexure
   _____ C. Splenic flexure
   _____ D. Jejunum

3. Which of the following is not supplied by the inferior mesenteric artery?
   _____ A. Sigmoid colon
   _____ B. Ascending colon
   _____ C. Transverse colon
   _____ D. Descending colon

4. Describe where the portal vein lies in relationship to the stomach and pancreas.

   _____

   _____

   _____

5. Which of the following structures is not considered retroperitoneal?
   _____ A. Ileum
   _____ B. Cecum
   _____ C. Descending colon
   _____ D. Kidneys

6. As the superior mesenteric vessels traverse through the head of the pancreas, is the artery or vein located farther to the right?

   _____

   _____

   _____

7. Describe the function and structure of the small intestine.

   _____

   _____

   _____

8. The stomach can be divided into three parts from superior to inferior:_____.

9. Describe the structure and function of the mesentery.

   _____

   _____

   _____

10. Which of the following would be located most anteriorly?
    _____ A. Jejunum
    _____ B. Spleen
    _____ C. Transverse colon
    _____ D. Pancreas

CLINICAL CORRELATIONS

■ Clinical Case 3-1

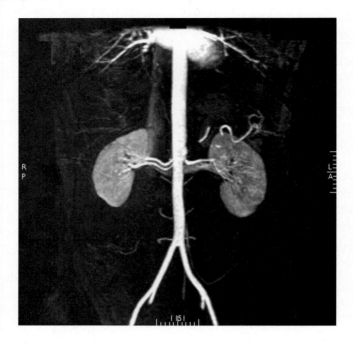

1. If this image was generated without radiation, which of the following would best describe the procedure:
   _____ A. Computed tomography angiography (CTA)
   _____ B. Magnetic resonance angiography (MRA)
   _____ C. Ultrasound
   _____ D. Positron emission tomography/computed tomography (PET/CT)

2. In this patient, the left renal artery originates from which of the following:
   _____ A. Right common iliac artery
   _____ B. Left common iliac artery
   _____ C. Abdominal aorta
   _____ D. Ascending aorta

3. How many renal arteries can be seen within this patient?
   _____ A. 1
   _____ B. 2
   _____ C. 3
   _____ D. 4

4. Which of the patient's kidneys appears to have stronger arterial blood flow?
   _____ A. Right
   _____ B. Left

5. A narrowing of the renal arteries would best be described by which of the following:
   _____ A. Dilation
   _____ B. Stenosis
   _____ C. Widening
   _____ D. Thinning

■ Clinical Case 3-2

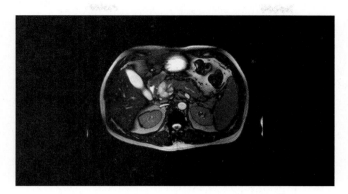

1. Describe the location of the inflammation found during magnetic resonance cholangiopancreatography of this 49-year-old male patient.

   _____

   _____

   _____

2. Describe the changes in adjacent tissues.

   _____

   _____

   _____

3. Describe the consistency, shape, and border.

   _____

   _____

   _____

■ Clinical Case 3-3

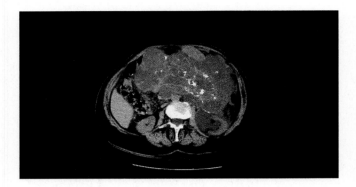

1. Describe the location of the mass found in this axial CT image of the abdomen.

   _____

   _____

   _____

2. Describe the changes in adjacent tissues.

   _____

   _____

   _____

3. Describe the consistency, shape, and border.

   _____

   _____

   _____

■ Clinical Case 3-4

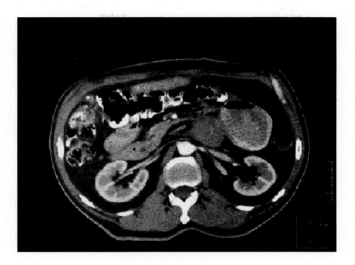

1. In this axial CT image, describe the location of the mass that a biopsy determined to be adenocarcinoma of the duodenum.

   _____

   _____

   _____

2. Describe the changes in adjacent tissues.

   _____

   _____

   _____

3. Describe the consistency, shape, and border.

   _____

   _____

   _____

■ Clinical Case 3-5

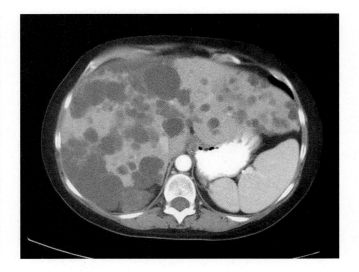

1. Describe the location of the autosomal dominant polycystic kidney disease in this axial CT image.

   _____

   _____

   _____

2. Describe the changes in adjacent tissues.

   _____

   _____

   _____

3. Describe the consistency, shape, and border.

   _____

   _____

   _____

■ Clinical Case 3-6

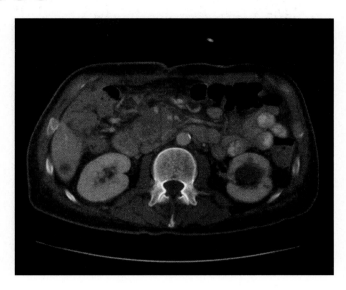

1. Describe the location of the pancreatic adenocarcinoma in this axial CT image of the upper abdomen.

   _____

   _____

   _____

2. Describe the changes in adjacent tissues.

   _____

   _____

   _____

3. Describe the consistency, shape, and border.

   _____

   _____

   _____

■ Clinical Case 3-7

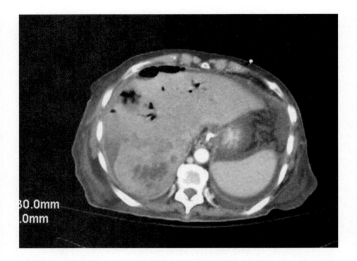

1. Describe the location of the liver abscess in this axial CT image of the upper abdomen.

_____

_____

_____

2. Describe the changes in adjacent tissues.

_____

_____

_____

3. Describe the consistency, shape, and border.

_____

_____

_____

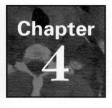

Male and Female Pelvis

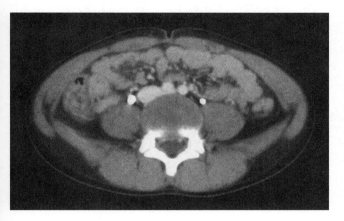

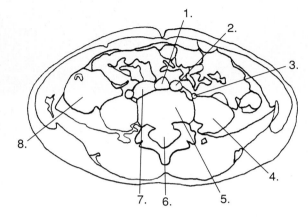

Figure 4-1

1. Which of the following is illustrated by 2?
   _____ A. Abdominal aorta
   _____ B. Inferior vena cava
   _____ C. Common iliac artery
   _____ D. Common iliac vein

2. Which of the following is illustrated by 6?
   _____ A. Intervertebral foramen
   _____ B. Vertebral foramen
   _____ C. Vertebral body
   _____ D. Intervertebral disk

3. Which number illustrates the psoas muscle?
   _____ A. 7
   _____ B. 8
   _____ C. 4
   _____ D. 1

4. Which of the following is illustrated by 7?
   _____ A. Common iliac vein
   _____ B. Common iliac artery
   _____ C. Abdominal aorta
   _____ D. Inferior vena cava

5. Which number illustrates the intervertebral disk?
   _____ A. 8
   _____ B. 5
   _____ C. 6
   _____ D. 4

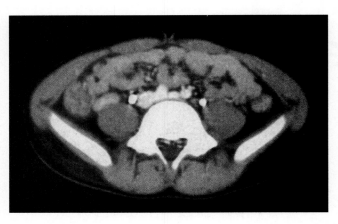 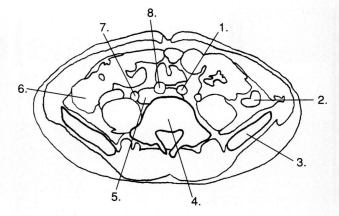

Figure 4-2

1. Which number illustrates the iliac crest?
   _____ A. 4
   _____ B. 2
   _____ C. 3
   _____ D. 1

2. Which of the following is illustrated by 8?
   _____ A. Inferior vena cava
   _____ B. Common iliac artery
   _____ C. Common iliac vein
   _____ D. Abdominal aorta

3. Which of the following is illustrated by 7?
   _____ A. Right ureter
   _____ B. Common iliac artery
   _____ C. Common iliac vein
   _____ D. Inferior mesenteric artery

4. Which number illustrates the inferior vena cava?
   _____ A. 8
   _____ B. 7
   _____ C. 1
   _____ D. 5

5. Which number illustrates the descending colon?
   _____ A. 5
   _____ B. 2
   _____ C. 7
   _____ D. 6

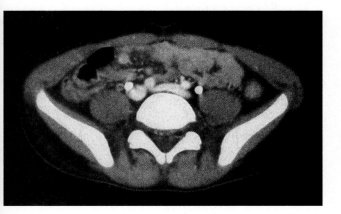
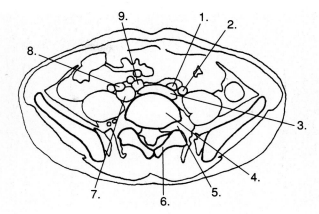

Figure 4-3

1. Which number illustrates the right common iliac artery?
   _____ A. 7
   _____ B. 2
   _____ C. 1
   _____ D. 9

2. Which of the following is illustrated by 7?
   _____ A. Left internal iliac vein
   _____ B. Right common iliac vein
   _____ C. Left external iliac artery
   _____ D. Right common iliac artery

3. Which of the following is illustrated by 3?
   _____ A. Abdominal aorta
   _____ B. Left common iliac artery
   _____ C. Inferior vena cava
   _____ D. Left common iliac vein

4. Which number illustrates the lamina?
   _____ A. 1
   _____ B. 5
   _____ C. 2
   _____ D. 6

5. Which of the following is illustrated by 8?
   _____ A. External iliac artery
   _____ B. Common iliac artery
   _____ C. Common iliac vein
   _____ D. Ureter

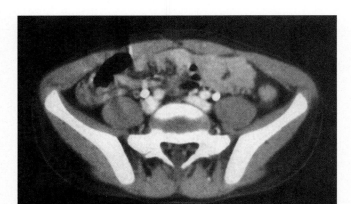

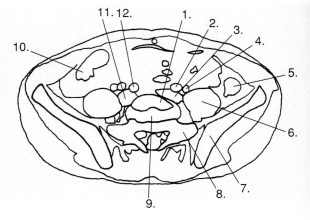

Figure 4-4

1. Which number illustrates the ilium?
   _____ A. 6
   _____ B. 5
   _____ C. 10
   _____ D. 7

2. Which of the following is illustrated by 1?
   _____ A. S1
   _____ B. L5
   _____ C. Intervertebral disk
   _____ D. L4

3. Which number illustrates the cecum?
   _____ A. 11
   _____ B. 7
   _____ C. 10
   _____ D. 5

4. Which of the following is illustrated by 2?
   _____ A. Left common iliac artery
   _____ B. Left common iliac vein
   _____ C. Left external iliac artery
   _____ D. Left external iliac vein

5. Which number illustrates the psoas muscle?
   _____ A. 7
   _____ B. 6
   _____ C. 5
   _____ D. 11

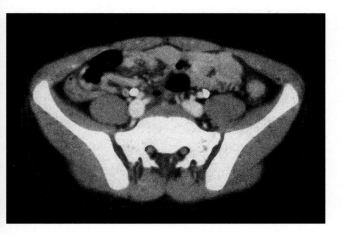
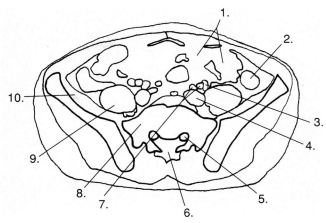

Figure 4-5

1. Which number illustrates the left common iliac vein?
   _____ A. 5
   _____ B. 7
   _____ C. 4
   _____ D. 3

2. Which of the following is illustrated by 10?
   _____ A. Loops of small bowel
   _____ B. Right ilium
   _____ C. Right iliacus muscle
   _____ D. Right psoas muscle

3. Which of the following is illustrated by 5?
   _____ A. Left ureter
   _____ B. Left vertebral foramen
   _____ C. Left common iliac vein
   _____ D. Sacral canal

4. Which number illustrates the left ureter?
   _____ A. 5
   _____ B. 3
   _____ C. 7
   _____ D. 2

5. Which number illustrates the psoas muscle?
   _____ A. 10
   _____ B. 4
   _____ C. 9
   _____ D. 6

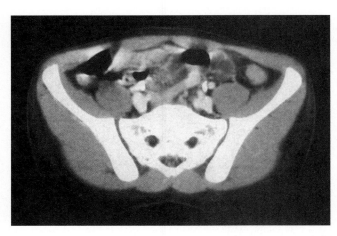

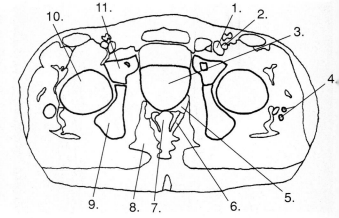

Figure 4-6

1. Which of the following is illustrated by 11?
   _____ A. Ileum
   _____ B. Cecum
   _____ C. Descending colon
   _____ D. Ascending colon

2. Which number illustrates the left internal iliac artery?
   _____ A. 5
   _____ B. 3
   _____ C. 4
   _____ D. 1

3. Which number illustrates the left external iliac artery?
   _____ A. 3
   _____ B. 4
   _____ C. 1
   _____ D. 5

4. Which of the following is illustrated by 2?
   _____ A. Jejunum
   _____ B. Ileum
   _____ C. Cecum
   _____ D. Descending colon

5. Which of the following is illustrated by 3?
   _____ A. Left common iliac vein
   _____ B. Left external iliac artery
   _____ C. Left internal iliac artery
   _____ D. Left ureter

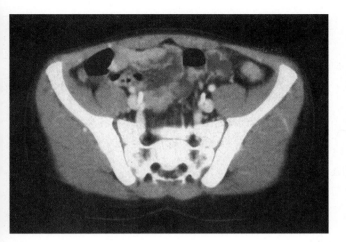 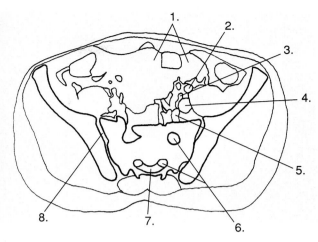

Figure 4-7

1. Which number illustrates the left common iliac vein?
   _____ A. 3
   _____ B. 2
   _____ C. 4
   _____ D. 5

2. Which of the following is illustrated by 7?
   _____ A. Left sacral foramen
   _____ B. Left internal iliac artery
   _____ C. Sacral canal
   _____ D. Intervertebral foramen

3. Which number illustrates the left sacral foramina?
   _____ A. 8
   _____ B. 7
   _____ C. 6
   _____ D. 5

4. Which of the following is illustrated by 5?
   _____ A. Left internal iliac artery
   _____ B. Left external iliac artery
   _____ C. Left common iliac vein
   _____ D. Left ureter

5. Which of the following is illustrated by 3?
   _____ A. Left external iliac artery
   _____ B. Left ureter
   _____ C. Left external iliac vein
   _____ D. Left internal iliac artery

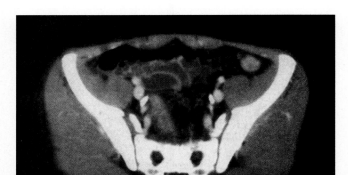 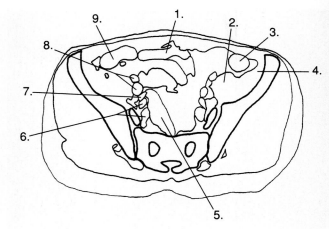

Figure 4-8

1. Which of the following is illustrated by 5?
   _____ A. Small bowel
   _____ B. Descending colon
   _____ C. Top of sigmoid colon
   _____ D. Top of bladder

2. Which number illustrates the external iliac artery and vein?
   _____ A. 9
   _____ B. 7
   _____ C. 8
   _____ D. 6

3. Which of the following is illustrated by 6?
   _____ A. Right common iliac artery and vein
   _____ B. Right external iliac artery and vein
   _____ C. Left external iliac artery and vein
   _____ D. Internal iliac artery and vein

4. Which number illustrates the iliacus muscle?
   _____ A. 3
   _____ B. 1
   _____ C. 2
   _____ D. 4

5. Which number illustrates the ureter?
   _____ A. 9
   _____ B. 8
   _____ C. 7
   _____ D. 6

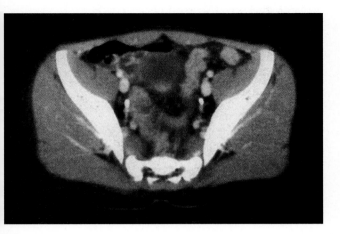
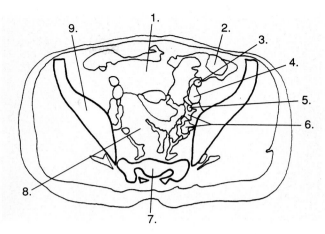

Figure 4-9

1. Which number illustrates the descending colon?
   _____ A. 8
   _____ B. 2
   _____ C. 1
   _____ D. 3

2. Which of the following is illustrated by 1?
   _____ A. Top of sigmoid colon
   _____ B. Top of bladder
   _____ C. Sacrum
   _____ D. Descending colon

3. Which of the following is illustrated by 4?
   _____ A. Left external iliac artery
   _____ B. Left ureter
   _____ C. Left common iliac artery
   _____ D. Left external iliac vein

4. Which number illustrates the left external iliac artery?
   _____ A. 4
   _____ B. 3
   _____ C. 5
   _____ D. 2

5. Which of the following is illustrated by 5?
   _____ A. Left ureter
   _____ B. Left external iliac artery
   _____ C. Left common iliac artery
   _____ D. Left external iliac vein

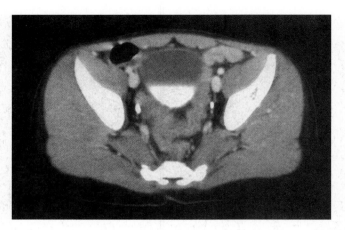
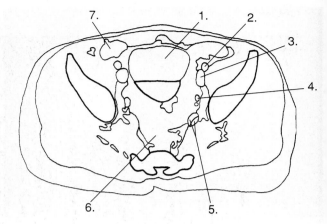

Figure 4-10

1. Which number illustrates the left external iliac artery?
   _____ A. 2
   _____ B. 5
   _____ C. 4
   _____ D. 3

2. Which of the following is illustrated by 6?
   _____ A. Bladder
   _____ B. Uterus
   _____ C. Sigmoid colon
   _____ D. Descending colon

3. Which number illustrates the left ureter?
   _____ A. 2
   _____ B. 5
   _____ C. 4
   _____ D. 3

4. Which of the following is illustrated by 1?
   _____ A. Small bowel
   _____ B. Bladder
   _____ C. Sigmoid colon
   _____ D. Descending colon

5. Which of the following is illustrated by 3?
   _____ A. Small bowel
   _____ B. Left ureter
   _____ C. Left external iliac artery
   _____ D. Left external iliac vein

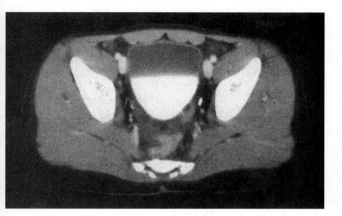
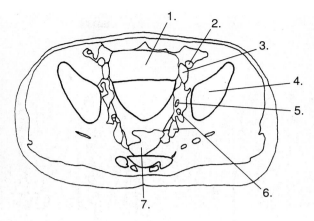

Figure 4-11

1. Which of the following is illustrated by 5?
   _____ A. Internal iliac vessel
   _____ B. External iliac vein
   _____ C. Ureter
   _____ D. External iliac artery

2. Which number illustrates the left external iliac artery?
   _____ A. 2
   _____ B. 5
   _____ C. 3
   _____ D. 6

3. Which of the following is illustrated by 7?
   _____ A. Rectum
   _____ B. Sigmoid colon
   _____ C. Descending colon
   _____ D. Seminal vesicles

4. Which of the following is illustrated by 4?
   _____ A. Pubic bone
   _____ B. Iliac bone
   _____ C. Ischial bone
   _____ D. Proximal femur

5. Which of the following is illustrated by 3?
   _____ A. Femoral artery
   _____ B. Ureter
   _____ C. External iliac artery
   _____ D. External iliac vein

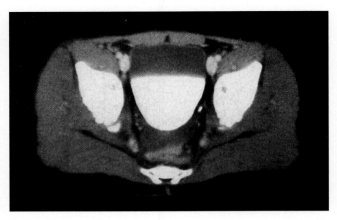 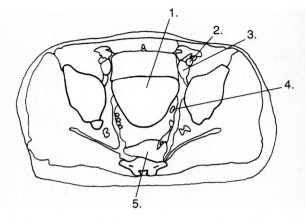

Figure 4-12

1. Which number illustrates the left external iliac vein?
   _____ A. 5
   _____ B. 3
   _____ C. 2
   _____ D. 4

2. Which of the following is illustrated by 5?
   _____ A. Rectum
   _____ B. Seminal vesicles
   _____ C. Sigmoid colon
   _____ D. Prostate gland

3. Which of the following is illustrated by 4?
   _____ A. Left seminal vesicle
   _____ B. Left ureter
   _____ C. Left external iliac artery
   _____ D. Left external iliac vein

4. Which number illustrates the bladder?
   _____ A. 1
   _____ B. 5
   _____ C. 4
   _____ D. 2

5. Which number illustrates the left external iliac artery?
   _____ A. 4
   _____ B. 2
   _____ C. 3
   _____ D. 1

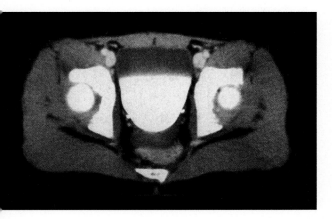
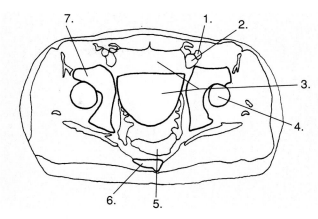

Figure 4-13

1. Which number illustrates the tip of the sacrum?
   _____ A. 2
   _____ B. 5
   _____ C. 4
   _____ D. 6

2. Which of the following is illustrated by 1?
   _____ A. External iliac vein
   _____ B. External iliac artery
   _____ C. Spermatic cord
   _____ D. Femoral artery

3. Which of the following is illustrated by 7?
   _____ A. Right ischium
   _____ B. Right ilium
   _____ C. Right pubis
   _____ D. Greater trochanter of femur

4. Which number illustrates the head of the femur?
   _____ A. 7
   _____ B. 4
   _____ C. 6
   _____ D. 1

5. Which number illustrates the external iliac artery?
   _____ A. 1
   _____ B. 2
   _____ C. 7
   _____ D. 5

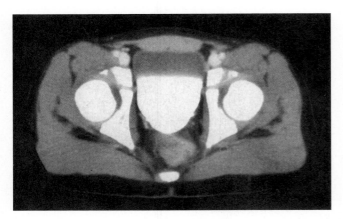 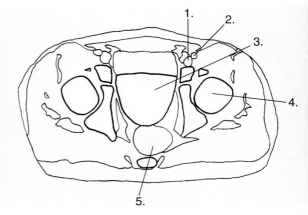

Figure 4-14

1. Which number illustrates the head of the femur?
   _____ A. 3
   _____ B. 2
   _____ C. 1
   _____ D. 4

2. Which of the following is illustrated by 4?
   _____ A. Head of right femur
   _____ B. Head of left femur
   _____ C. Right ilium
   _____ D. Left ilium

3. Which number illustrates the femoral artery?
   _____ A. 3
   _____ B. 2
   _____ C. 4
   _____ D. 1

4. Which of the following is illustrated by 1?
   _____ A. Right external iliac vein
   _____ B. Left external iliac vein
   _____ C. Right femoral vein
   _____ D. Left femoral vein

5. Which of the following is illustrated by 5?
   _____ A. Seminal vesicles
   _____ B. Sigmoid colon
   _____ C. Rectum
   _____ D. Bladder

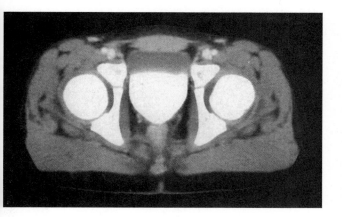 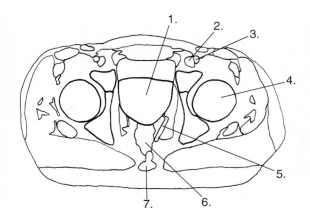

Figure 4-15

1. Which of the following is illustrated by 2?
   _____ A. Right external iliac vein
   _____ B. Left femoral vein
   _____ C. Left external iliac vein
   _____ D. Right femoral vein

2. Which number illustrates the coccyx?
   _____ A. 5
   _____ B. 2
   _____ C. 1
   _____ D. 7

3. Which number illustrates the pelvic diaphragm?
   _____ A. 1
   _____ B. 6
   _____ C. 5
   _____ D. 3

4. Which of the following is illustrated by 1?
   _____ A. Coccyx
   _____ B. Head of the left femur
   _____ C. Bladder
   _____ D. Rectum

5. Which number illustrates the rectum?
   _____ A. 5
   _____ B. 7
   _____ C. 6
   _____ D. 1

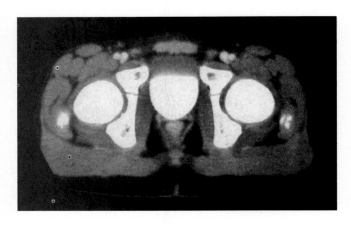
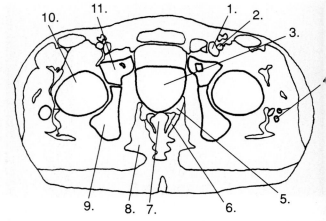

Figure 4-16

1. Which of the following is illustrated by 9?
   _____ A. Right pubis
   _____ B. Right ileum
   _____ C. Right ischium
   _____ D. Right ilium

2. Which number illustrates the pelvic diaphragm?
   _____ A. 5
   _____ B. 7
   _____ C. 8
   _____ D. 6

3. Which of the following is illustrated by 1?
   _____ A. Femoral vein
   _____ B. Femoral artery
   _____ C. External iliac artery
   _____ D. External iliac vein

4. Which number illustrates the pubis?
   _____ A. 10
   _____ B. 9
   _____ C. 11
   _____ D. 3

5. Which number illustrates the seminal vesicle?
   _____ A. 7
   _____ B. 6
   _____ C. 5
   _____ D. 8

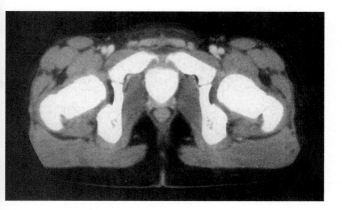 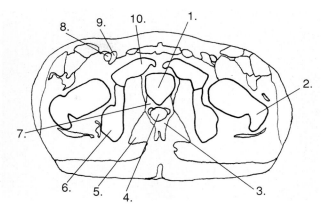

Figure 4-17

1. Which number illustrates the right femoral vein?
   _____ A. 8
   _____ B. 6
   _____ C. 4
   _____ D. 9

2. Which of the following is illustrated by 7?
   _____ A. Seminal vesicle
   _____ B. Adnexal area
   _____ C. Prostate
   _____ D. Ischiorectal fossa

3. Which number illustrates the bladder?
   _____ A. 1
   _____ B. 7
   _____ C. 3
   _____ D. 4

4. Which of the following is illustrated by 6?
   _____ A. Pubis
   _____ B. Ileum
   _____ C. Ischium
   _____ D. Ilium

5. Which of the following is illustrated by 4?
   _____ A. Pelvic diaphragm
   _____ B. Rectum
   _____ C. Bladder
   _____ D. Sigmoid colon

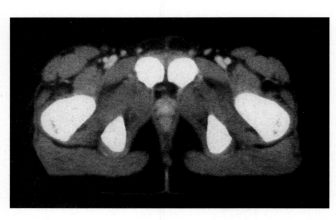
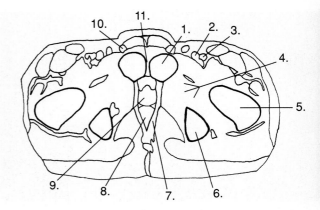

Figure 4-18

1. Which of the following is illustrated by 6?
   _____ A. Ischial tuberosity
   _____ B. Pubic bone
   _____ C. Ischial spine
   _____ D. Proximal femur

2. Which of the following is illustrated by 1?
   _____ A. Ilium
   _____ B. Pubic bone
   _____ C. Ischial spine
   _____ D. Ischial tuberosity

3. Which number illustrates the prostate?
   _____ A. 6
   _____ B. 8
   _____ C. 1
   _____ D. 9

4. Which number illustrates the femoral artery?
   _____ A. 10
   _____ B. 2
   _____ C. 3
   _____ D. 1

5. Which of the following is illustrated by 5?
   _____ A. Neck of the left femur
   _____ B. Greater trochanter of femur
   _____ C. Lesser trochanter of femur
   _____ D. Ischial bone

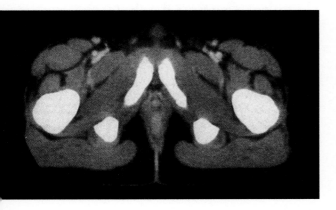
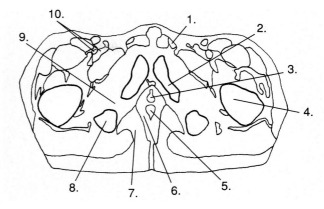

Figure 4-19

1. Which of the following is illustrated by 6?
   _____ A. Pelvic diaphragm
   _____ B. Obturator foramina
   _____ C. Ischiorectal fossa
   _____ D. Prostate

2. Which number illustrates the ischial tuberosity?
   _____ A. 9
   _____ B. 2
   _____ C. 8
   _____ D. 4

3. Which number illustrates the spermatic cord?
   _____ A. 1
   _____ B. 5
   _____ C. 10
   _____ D. 3

4. Which of the following is illustrated by 2?
   _____ A. Superior pubic ramus
   _____ B. Interior pubic ramus
   _____ C. Ischial tuberosity
   _____ D. Ischial ramus

5. Which number illustrates the prostate?
   _____ A. 6
   _____ B. 3
   _____ C. 5
   _____ D. 2

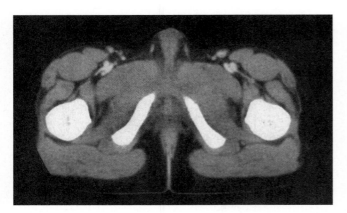 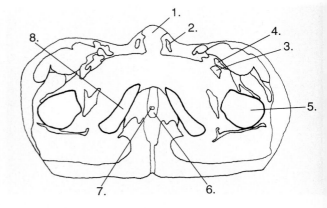

Figure 4-20

1. Which of the following is illustrated by 1?
   _____ A. Corpus spongiosum
   _____ B. Corpus cavernosum
   _____ C. Urethra
   _____ D. Symphysis pubis

2. Which number illustrates the urethra?
   _____ A. 5
   _____ B. 2
   _____ C. 7
   _____ D. 1

3. Which number illustrates the ischial ramus?
   _____ A. 5
   _____ B. 2
   _____ C. 1
   _____ D. 8

4. Which of the following is illustrated by 2?
   _____ A. Femoral artery
   _____ B. Femoral vein
   _____ C. Spermatic cord
   _____ D. Urethra

5. Which of the following is illustrated by 6?
   _____ A. Corpus cavernosum
   _____ B. Left spermatic cord
   _____ C. Urethra
   _____ D. Corpus spongiosum

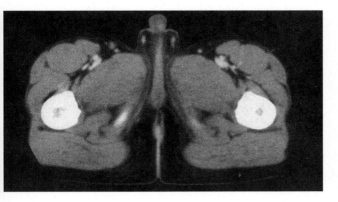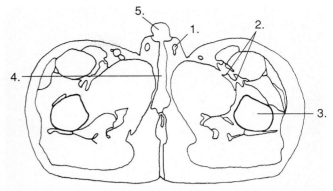

Figure 4-21

1. Which number illustrates the corpus spongiosum?
   _____ A. 5
   _____ B. 2
   _____ C. 4
   _____ D. 1

2. Which of the following is illustrated by 1?
   _____ A. Femoral artery
   _____ B. Spermatic cord
   _____ C. Femoral vein
   _____ D. External iliac artery

3. Which number illustrates the corpus cavernosum?
   _____ A. 3
   _____ B. 1
   _____ C. 4
   _____ D. 5

4. Which of the following is illustrated by 2?
   _____ A. Femoral vessels
   _____ B. Corpus spongiosum
   _____ C. Spermatic cord
   _____ D. External iliac vessels

5. Which of the following is illustrated by 3?
   _____ A. Ischial tuberosity
   _____ B. Head of femur
   _____ C. Shaft of the left femur
   _____ D. Greater trochanter of femur

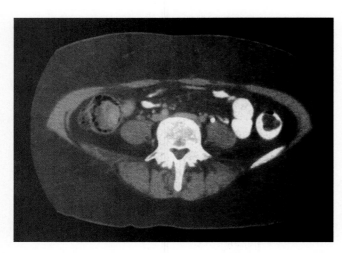
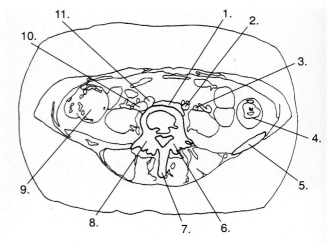

Figure 4-22

1. Which number illustrates the pedicle of L5?
   _____ A. 8
   _____ B. 6
   _____ C. 7
   _____ D. 9

2. Which of the following is illustrated by 2?
   _____ A. Ureter
   _____ B. Internal iliac vein
   _____ C. Common iliac artery
   _____ D. Common iliac vein

3. Which number illustrates the left common iliac vein?
   _____ A. 11
   _____ B. 2
   _____ C. 1
   _____ D. 3

4. Which of the following is illustrated by 6?
   _____ A. Intervertebral foramen
   _____ B. Lamina of L5
   _____ C. Spinous process of L5
   _____ D. Pedicle of L5

5. Which of the following is illustrated by 3?
   _____ A. Common iliac vein
   _____ B. Common iliac artery
   _____ C. External iliac artery
   _____ D. Ureter

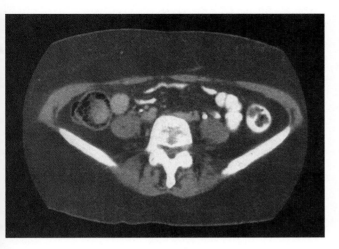
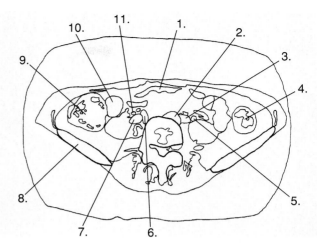

Figure 4-23

1. Which of the following is illustrated by 4?
   _____ A. Descending colon
   _____ B. Ascending colon
   _____ C. Ileum
   _____ D. Cecum

2. Which number illustrates the left common iliac artery?
   _____ A. 5
   _____ B. 2
   _____ C. 3
   _____ D. 6

3. Which of the following is illustrated by 1?
   _____ A. Cecum
   _____ B. Transverse colon
   _____ C. Small bowel
   _____ D. Sigmoid colon

4. Which number illustrates the right common iliac vein?
   _____ A. 10
   _____ B. 7
   _____ C. 11
   _____ D. 6

5. Which of the following is illustrated by 11?
   _____ A. Ureter
   _____ B. Common iliac vein
   _____ C. External iliac artery
   _____ D. Common iliac artery

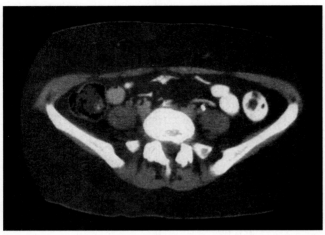 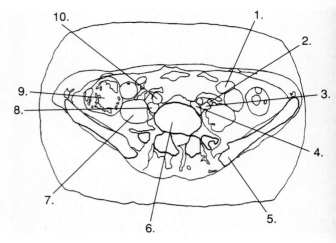

Figure 4-24

1. Which of the following is illustrated by 2?
   _____ A. Common iliac vein
   _____ B. Ureter
   _____ C. Common iliac artery
   _____ D. External iliac artery

2. Which number illustrates the right common iliac artery?
   _____ A. 3
   _____ B. 8
   _____ C. 2
   _____ D. 10

3. Which number illustrates the left common iliac artery?
   _____ A. 2
   _____ B. 3
   _____ C. 4
   _____ D. 10

4. Which number illustrates the left common iliac vein?
   _____ A. 3
   _____ B. 2
   _____ C. 1
   _____ D. 4

5. Which of the following is illustrated by 10?
   _____ A. Common iliac vein
   _____ B. Psoas muscle
   _____ C. Common iliac artery
   _____ D. Inferior mesenteric artery

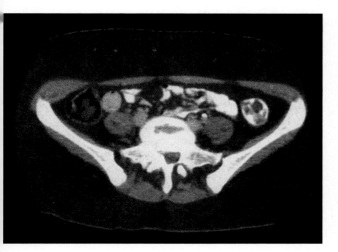
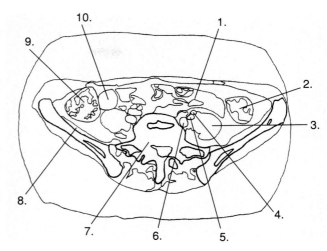

Figure 4-25

1. Which number illustrates the small bowel?
   _____ A. 1
   _____ B. 3
   _____ C. 2
   _____ D. 9

2. Which of the following is illustrated by 4?
   _____ A. Common iliac artery
   _____ B. Ureter
   _____ C. Common iliac vein
   _____ D. External iliac artery

3. Which of the following is illustrated by 8?
   _____ A. Psoas muscle
   _____ B. Iliacus muscle
   _____ C. Ileum
   _____ D. Ilium

4. Which number illustrates the common iliac artery?
   _____ A. 6
   _____ B. 3
   _____ C. 5
   _____ D. 4

5. Which number illustrates the descending colon?
   _____ A. 2
   _____ B. 9
   _____ C. 10
   _____ D. 3

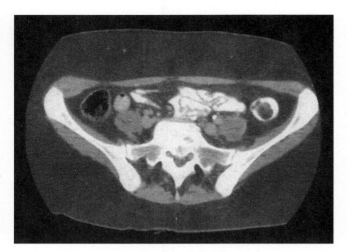

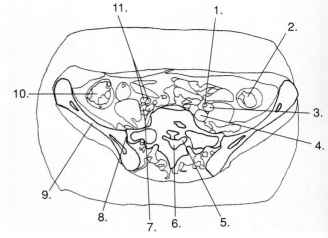

Figure 4-26

1. Which number illustrates the right sacroiliac joint?
   _____ A. 9
   _____ B. 5
   _____ C. 8
   _____ D. 6

2. Which of the following is illustrated by 4?
   _____ A. Common iliac vein
   _____ B. Ureter
   _____ C. Internal iliac artery
   _____ D. Common iliac artery

3. Which of the following is illustrated by 3?
   _____ A. Internal iliac artery
   _____ B. Common iliac artery
   _____ C. Ureter
   _____ D. External iliac vein

4. Which number illustrates the cecum?
   _____ A. 2
   _____ B. 9
   _____ C. 4
   _____ D. 10

5. Which number illustrates the descending colon?
   _____ A. 10
   _____ B. 6
   _____ C. 3
   _____ D. 2

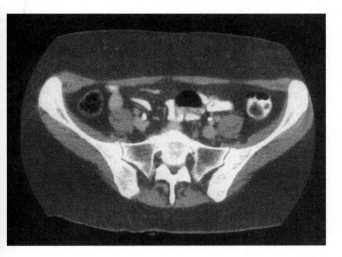
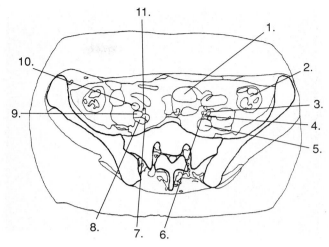

Figure 4-27

1. Which of the following is illustrated by 6?
   _____ A. External iliac artery
   _____ B. Internal iliac artery
   _____ C. Internal iliac vein
   _____ D. Ureter

2. Which number illustrates the right external iliac artery?
   _____ A. 11
   _____ B. 8
   _____ C. 10
   _____ D. 7

3. Which of the following illustrates the right internal iliac vein?
   _____ A. 9
   _____ B. 8
   _____ C. 7
   _____ D. 10

4. Which number illustrates the left common iliac vein?
   _____ A. 6
   _____ B. 4
   _____ C. 5
   _____ D. 3

5. Which of the following illustrates the left external iliac artery?
   _____ A. 5
   _____ B. 4
   _____ C. 3
   _____ D. 6

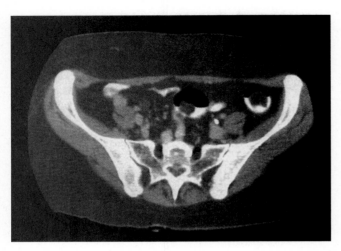 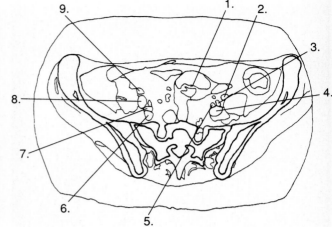

Figure 4-28

1. Which of the following is illustrated by 8?
   _____ A. External iliac vein
   _____ B. Internal iliac vein
   _____ C. External iliac artery
   _____ D. Internal iliac artery

2. Which number illustrates the external iliac artery?
   _____ A. 2
   _____ B. 4
   _____ C. 3
   _____ D. 5

3. Which of the following is illustrated by 5?
   _____ A. Common iliac vein
   _____ B. Ureter
   _____ C. Internal iliac artery
   _____ D. External iliac artery

4. Which number illustrates the internal iliac artery?
   _____ A. 8
   _____ B. 7
   _____ C. 6
   _____ D. 9

5. Which of the following is illustrated by 3?
   _____ A. Ureter
   _____ B. External iliac artery
   _____ C. Common iliac vein
   _____ D. Internal iliac artery

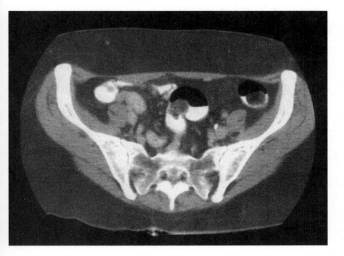

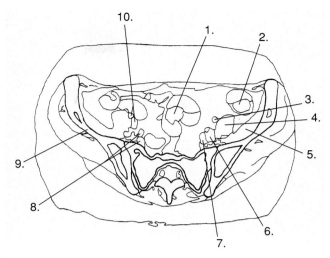

Figure 4-29

1. Which of the following is illustrated by 2?
   _____ A. Descending colon
   _____ B. Sigmoid colon
   _____ C. Left psoas muscle
   _____ D. Ascending colon

2. Which number illustrates the left internal iliac artery?
   _____ A. 6
   _____ B. 3
   _____ C. 4
   _____ D. 7

3. Which number illustrates the iliacus muscle?
   _____ A. 4
   _____ B. 2
   _____ C. 5
   _____ D. 6

4. Which of the following is illustrated by 4?
   _____ A. Small bowel
   _____ B. Psoas muscle
   _____ C. Internal iliac vein
   _____ D. Sigmoid colon

5. Which of the following is illustrated by 6?
   _____ A. External iliac artery
   _____ B. Internal iliac artery
   _____ C. Internal iliac vein
   _____ D. Common iliac vein

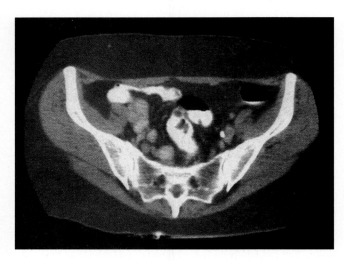
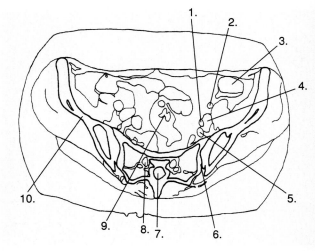

Figure 4-30

1. Which of the following is illustrated by 4?
   _____ A. External iliac artery
   _____ B. Common iliac vein
   _____ C. Ureter
   _____ D. Internal iliac artery

2. Which number illustrates the sigmoid colon?
   _____ A. 6
   _____ B. 5
   _____ C. 8
   _____ D. 9

3. Which of the following is illustrated by 5?
   _____ A. Internal iliac artery
   _____ B. Ureter
   _____ C. Common iliac vein
   _____ D. External iliac artery

4. Which number illustrates the sacral canal?
   _____ A. 7
   _____ B. 9
   _____ C. 8
   _____ D. 10

5. Which number illustrates the sacral foramen?
   _____ A. 10
   _____ B. 7
   _____ C. 8
   _____ D. 6

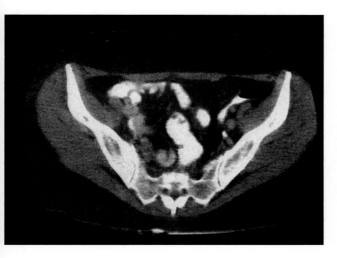 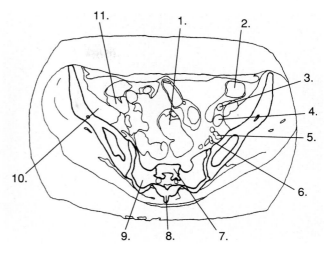

Figure 4-31

1. Which of the following is illustrated by 9?
   _____ A. Lateral part of the sacrum
   _____ B. Spinous process
   _____ C. Vertebral body
   _____ D. Sigmoid colon

2. Which number illustrates the psoas muscle?
   _____ A. 10
   _____ B. 9
   _____ C. 1
   _____ D. 11

3. Which of the following is illustrated by 5?
   _____ A. External iliac artery
   _____ B. Internal iliac vein
   _____ C. External iliac vein
   _____ D. Internal iliac artery

4. Which number illustrates the spinous process?
   _____ A. 9
   _____ B. 8
   _____ C. 7
   _____ D. 11

5. Which of the following illustrates the iliacus muscle?
   _____ A. 11
   _____ B. 9
   _____ C. 10
   _____ D. 8

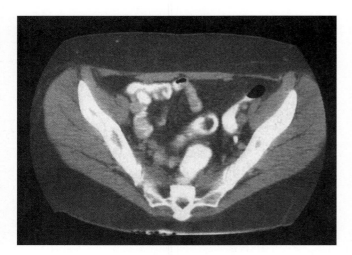
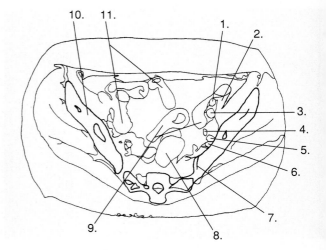

Figure 4-32

1. Which of the following is illustrated by 8?
   _____ A. Ileum
   _____ B. Rectum
   _____ C. Sigmoid colon
   _____ D. Uterus

2. Which number illustrates the left internal iliac artery?
   _____ A. 5
   _____ B. 6
   _____ C. 3
   _____ D. 1

3. Which of the following is illustrated by 4?
   _____ A. Internal iliac vein
   _____ B. Internal iliac artery
   _____ C. External iliac vein
   _____ D. Ureter

4. Which number illustrates the sigmoid colon?
   _____ A. 8
   _____ B. 7
   _____ C. 9
   _____ D. 11

5. Which of the following is illustrated by 1?
   _____ A. External iliac artery
   _____ B. Internal iliac vein
   _____ C. Internal iliac artery
   _____ D. External iliac vein

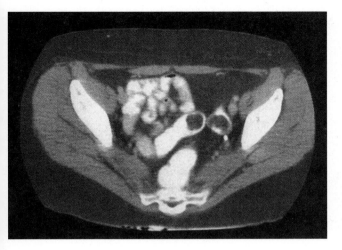

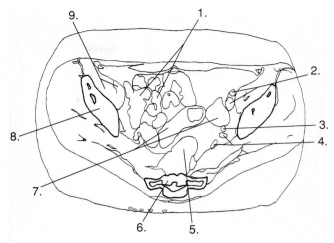

Figure 4-33

1. Which of the following is illustrated by 9?
   _____ A.   Loops of the ileum
   _____ B.   Iliac muscle
   _____ C.   Iliopsoas muscle
   _____ D.   Psoas muscle

2. Which number illustrates the rectum?
   _____ A.   5
   _____ B.   9
   _____ C.   1
   _____ D.   7

3. Which of the following is illustrated by 6?
   _____ A.   Ilium
   _____ B.   Ischium
   _____ C.   Coccyx
   _____ D.   Sacrum

4. Which of the following is illustrated by 7?
   _____ A.   Descending colon
   _____ B.   Rectum
   _____ C.   Loops of the ileum
   _____ D.   Sigmoid colon

5. Which number illustrates the ilium?
   _____ A.   5
   _____ B.   1
   _____ C.   8
   _____ D.   9

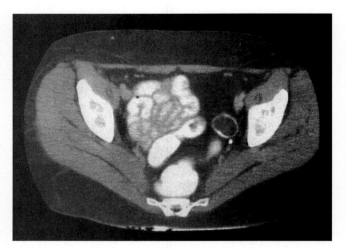
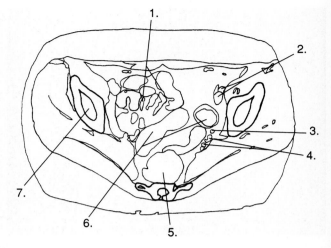

Figure 4-34

1. Which of the following is illustrated by 2?
   _____ A. Femoral artery and vein
   _____ B. External iliac artery and vein
   _____ C. Gluteal artery and vein
   _____ D. Internal iliac artery and vein

2. Which number illustrates the sigmoid colon?
   _____ A. 4
   _____ B. 1
   _____ C. 5
   _____ D. 6

3. Which number illustrates the left internal iliac artery
   and vein?
   _____ A. 2
   _____ B. 4
   _____ C. 3
   _____ D. 6

4. Which of the following is illustrated by 1?
   _____ A. Sigmoid colon
   _____ B. Top of bladder
   _____ C. Loops of ileum
   _____ D. Loops of ilium

5. Which number illustrates the rectum?
   _____ A. 7
   _____ B. 5
   _____ C. 6
   _____ D. 3

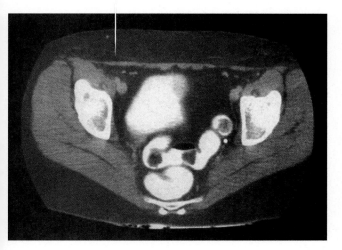

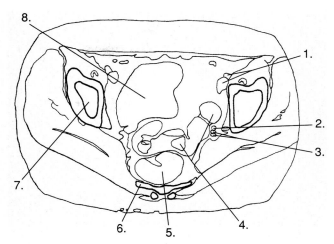

Figure 4-35

1. Which of the following is illustrated by 7?
   _____ A. Ischium
   _____ B. Pubis
   _____ C. Ilium
   _____ D. Ileum

2. Which of the following is illustrated by 4?
   _____ A. Small bowel
   _____ B. Sigmoid colon
   _____ C. Descending colon
   _____ D. Rectum

3. Which number illustrates the rectum?
   _____ A. 6
   _____ B. 5
   _____ C. 4
   _____ D. 8

4. Which of the following illustrates the bladder?
   _____ A. 5
   _____ B. 4
   _____ C. 7
   _____ D. 8

5. Which of the following is illustrated by 3?
   _____ A. Gluteal artery and vein
   _____ B. Common iliac artery and vein
   _____ C. External iliac artery and vein
   _____ D. Internal iliac artery and vein

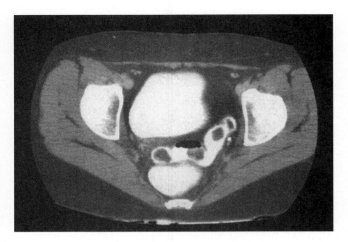 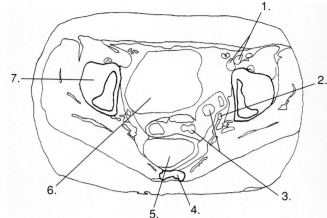

Figure 4-36

1. Which of the following is illustrated by 7?
   _____ A. Ileum
   _____ B. Ilium
   _____ C. Ischium
   _____ D. Pubis

2. Which of the following is illustrated by 2?
   _____ A. External iliac artery
   _____ B. Internal iliac artery
   _____ C. Ureter
   _____ D. Internal iliac vein

3. Which of the following is illustrated by 3?
   _____ A. Sigmoid colon
   _____ B. Rectum
   _____ C. Small bowel
   _____ D. Descending colon

4. Which number illustrates the rectum?
   _____ A. 2
   _____ B. 6
   _____ C. 5
   _____ D. 3

5. Which number illustrates the bladder?
   _____ A. 5
   _____ B. 6
   _____ C. 3
   _____ D. 2

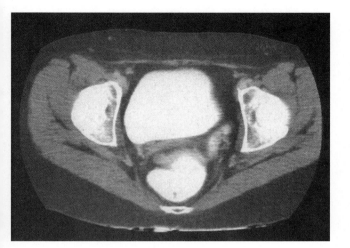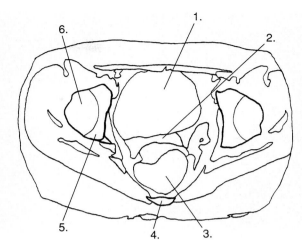

Figure 4-37

1. Which of the following is illustrated by 2?
   _____ A. Cervix of uterus
   _____ B. Vagina
   _____ C. Adnexal area
   _____ D. Fundus of uterus

2. Which of the following is illustrated by 4?
   _____ A. Sacrum
   _____ B. Coccyx
   _____ C. Ischium
   _____ D. Pubis

3. Which of the following is illustrated by 5?
   _____ A. Ilium
   _____ B. Ischium
   _____ C. Pubis
   _____ D. Femur

4. Which of the following is illustrated by 3?
   _____ A. Sigmoid colon
   _____ B. Rectum
   _____ C. Vagina
   _____ D. Cervix of uterus

5. Which of the following is illustrated by 6?
   _____ A. Shaft of femur
   _____ B. Ilium
   _____ C. Neck of femur
   _____ D. Head of femur

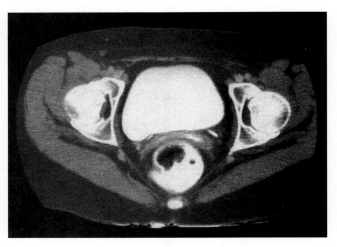

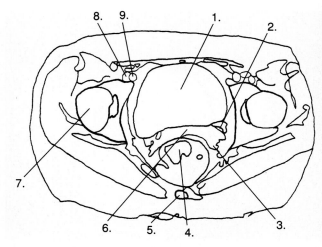

Figure 4-38

1. Which of the following is illustrated by 3?
   _____ A. Adnexal area
   _____ B. Pelvic diaphragm
   _____ C. Body of uterus
   _____ D. Seminal vesicle

2. Which number illustrates the femoral artery?
   _____ A. 2
   _____ B. 9
   _____ C. 8
   _____ D. 5

3. Which number illustrates the femoral vein?
   _____ A. 3
   _____ B. 8
   _____ C. 9
   _____ D. 7

4. Which of the following is illustrated by 2?
   _____ A. Internal iliac artery
   _____ B. Ureter
   _____ C. Femoral nerve
   _____ D. Internal iliac vein

5. Which of the following is illustrated by 5?
   _____ A. Ilium
   _____ B. Ischium
   _____ C. Sacrum
   _____ D. Coccyx

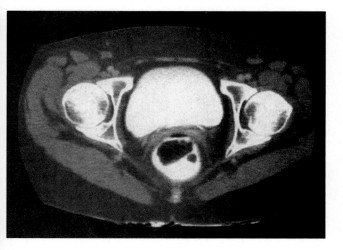 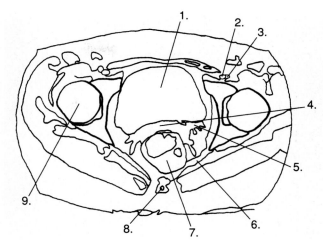

Figure 4-39

1. Which number illustrates the femoral vein?
    _____ A. 8
    _____ B. 2
    _____ C. 3
    _____ D. 9

2. Which of the following is illustrated by 7?
    _____ A. Left adnexal area
    _____ B. Body of the uterus
    _____ C. Bladder
    _____ D. Rectum

3. Which of the following is illustrated by 3?
    _____ A. Femoral vein
    _____ B. Femoral artery
    _____ C. External iliac artery
    _____ D. External iliac vein

4. Which number illustrates the pelvic diaphragm?
    _____ A. 4
    _____ B. 7
    _____ C. 6
    _____ D. 5

5. Which of the following is illustrated by 5?
    _____ A. Adnexal area
    _____ B. Body of uterus
    _____ C. Pelvic diaphragm
    _____ D. Ureter

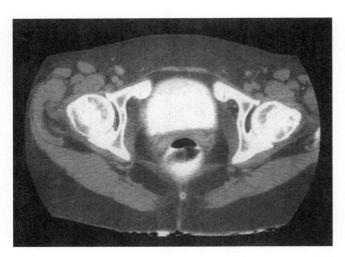 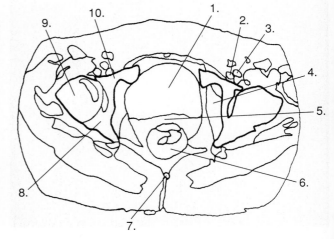

Figure 4-40

1. Which of the following is illustrated by 4?
   _____ A. Left adnexal area
   _____ B. Body of uterus
   _____ C. Pelvic diaphragm
   _____ D. Obturator foramen

2. Which number illustrates the pubis?
   _____ A. 5
   _____ B. 9
   _____ C. 8
   _____ D. 10

3. Which of the following is illustrated by 9?
   _____ A. Right pubis
   _____ B. Head of right femur
   _____ C. Right ischium
   _____ D. Greater trochanter of femur

4. Which of the following is illustrated by 7?
   _____ A. Coccyx
   _____ B. Sacrum
   _____ C. Ischium
   _____ D. Pubis

5. Which number illustrates the ischium?
   _____ A. 4
   _____ B. 9
   _____ C. 8
   _____ D. 5

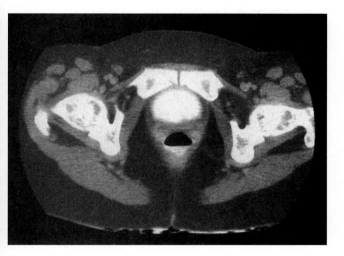
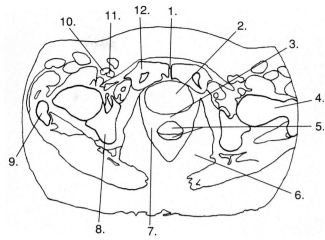

Figure 4-41

1. Which number illustrates the pubis?
   _____ A. 9
   _____ B. 8
   _____ C. 1
   _____ D. 12

2. Which of the following is illustrated by 1?
   _____ A. Right pubis
   _____ B. Left ischiorectal fossa
   _____ C. Symphysis pubis
   _____ D. Obturator foramen

3. Which number illustrates the pelvic diaphragm?
   _____ A. 1
   _____ B. 6
   _____ C. 3
   _____ D. 7

4. Which of the following is illustrated by 3?
   _____ A. Cervix of uterus
   _____ B. Body of uterus
   _____ C. Pelvic diaphragm
   _____ D. Left ischiorectal fossa

5. Which number illustrates the ischiorectal fossa?
   _____ A. 4
   _____ B. 8
   _____ C. 7
   _____ D. 6

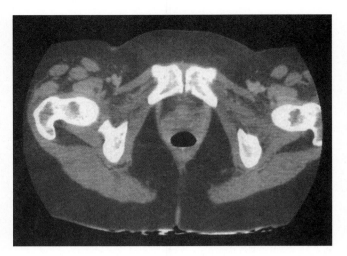 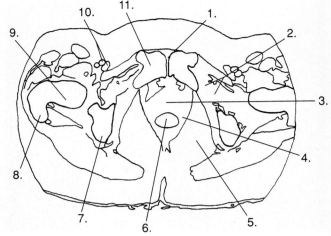

Figure 4-42

1. Which of the following is illustrated by 2?
   _____ A. Symphysis pubis
   _____ B. Pelvic diaphragm
   _____ C. Obturator foramen
   _____ D. Ischiorectal fossa

2. Which number illustrates the ischial tuberosity?
   _____ A. 9
   _____ B. 7
   _____ C. 8
   _____ D. 6

3. Which number illustrates the ischiorectal fossa?
   _____ A. 2
   _____ B. 4
   _____ C. 3
   _____ D. 5

4. Which of the following is illustrated by 8?
   _____ A. Greater trochanter of right femur
   _____ B. Neck of right femur
   _____ C. Lesser trochanter of right femur
   _____ D. Right ischial tuberosity

5. Which of the following is illustrated by 3?
   _____ A. Body of uterus
   _____ B. Adnexal area
   _____ C. Cervix of uterus
   _____ D. Pelvic diaphragm

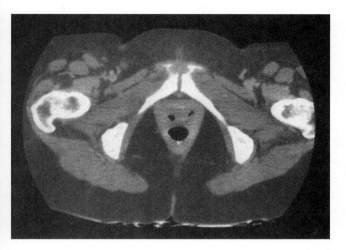
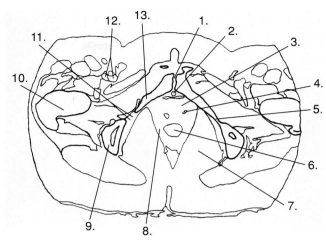

Figure 4-43

1. Which number illustrates the cervix of the uterus?
   _____ A. 4
   _____ B. 3
   _____ C. 2
   _____ D. 6

2. Which of the following is illustrated by 2?
   _____ A. Urethra
   _____ B. Posterior vaginal fornix
   _____ C. Ureter
   _____ D. Cervix of uterus

3. Which number illustrates the obturator foramen?
   _____ A. 1
   _____ B. 2
   _____ C. 11
   _____ D. 7

4. Which of the following is illustrated by 5?
   _____ A. Ischial ramus
   _____ B. Ischial tuberosity
   _____ C. Superior pubic ramus
   _____ D. Inferior pubic ramus

5. Which of the following is illustrated by 4?
   _____ A. Symphysis pubis
   _____ B. Posterior vaginal fornix
   _____ C. Pelvic diaphragm
   _____ D. Urethra

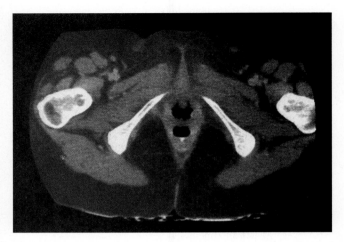
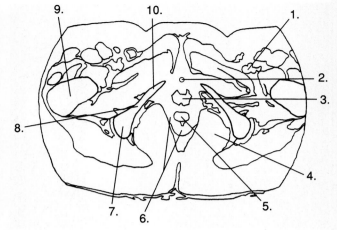

Figure 4-44

1. Which of the following is illustrated by 1?
   _____ A. Left ischiorectal fossa
   _____ B. Left adnexal area
   _____ C. Contents of femoral sheath
   _____ D. External iliac vessels

2. Which of the following is illustrated by 9?
   _____ A. Ischial ramus
   _____ B. Pubic ramus
   _____ C. Shaft of femur
   _____ D. Ischial tuberosity

3. Which of the following is illustrated by 3?
   _____ A. Vagina
   _____ B. Rectum
   _____ C. Urethra
   _____ D. Opening within uterus

4. Which of the following is illustrated by 8?
   _____ A. Ilium
   _____ B. Ischial tuberosity
   _____ C. Pubic ramus
   _____ D. Ischial ramus

5. Which number illustrates the ischial tuberosity?
   _____ A. 7
   _____ B. 8
   _____ C. 10
   _____ D. 9

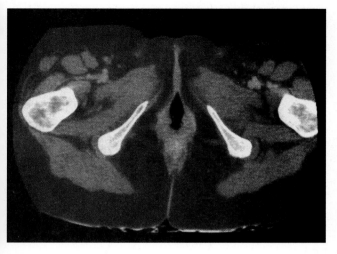 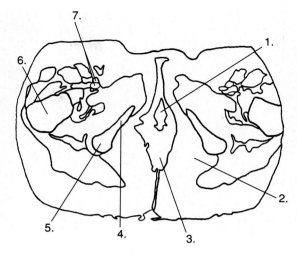

Figure 4-45

1. Which of the following is illustrated by 2?
    _____ A. Pelvic diaphragm
    _____ B. Ischiorectal fossa
    _____ C. Ischial tuberosity
    _____ D. Femoral sheath

2. Which number illustrates the ischial tuberosity?
    _____ A. 4
    _____ B. 1
    _____ C. 5
    _____ D. 6

3. Which of the following is illustrated by 1?
    _____ A. Vagina
    _____ B. Rectum
    _____ C. Opening within uterus
    _____ D. Ischiorectal fossa

4. Which number illustrates the pelvic diaphragm?
    _____ A. 2
    _____ B. 3
    _____ C. 6
    _____ D. 5

5. Which number illustrates the ischial ramus?
    _____ A. 4
    _____ B. 5
    _____ C. 7
    _____ D. 6

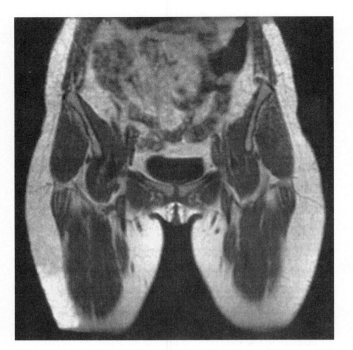
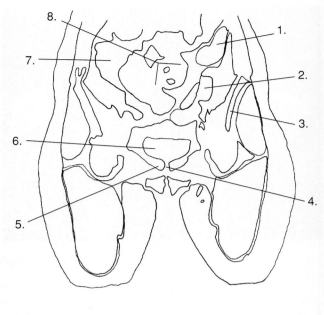

Figure 4-46

1. Which of the following is illustrated by 5?
_____ A. Ilium
_____ B. Ischium
_____ C. Pubis
_____ D. Ileum

2. Which of the following is illustrated by 7?
_____ A. Cecum
_____ B. Ascending colon
_____ C. Descending colon
_____ D. Sigmoid colon

3. Which of the following is illustrated by 2?
_____ A. Cecum
_____ B. Ascending colon
_____ C. Descending colon
_____ D. Sigmoid colon

4. Which number illustrates the descending colon?
_____ A. 7
_____ B. 2
_____ C. 1
_____ D. 8

5. Which number illustrates the ilium?
_____ A. 5
_____ B. 4
_____ C. 3
_____ D. 8

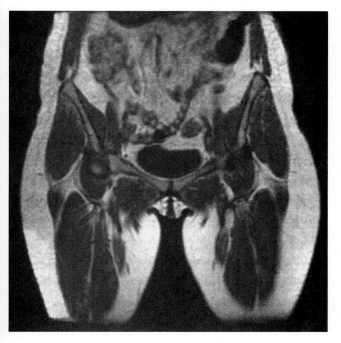
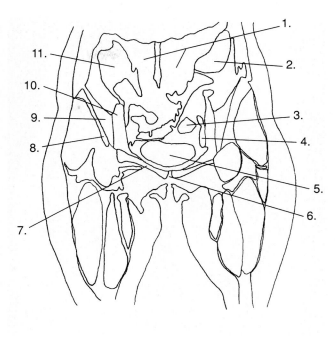

Figure 4-47

1. Which of the following is illustrated by 2?
   _____ A. Cecum
   _____ B. Descending colon
   _____ C. Sigmoid colon
   _____ D. Small bowel

2. Which of the following is illustrated by 3?
   _____ A. Sigmoid colon
   _____ B. Small bowel
   _____ C. Descending colon
   _____ D. Cecum

3. Which number illustrates the psoas muscle?
   _____ A. 4
   _____ B. 8
   _____ C. 9
   _____ D. 10

4. Which of the following is illustrated by 4?
   _____ A. Internal iliac artery and vein
   _____ B. External iliac artery and vein
   _____ C. Femoral artery and vein
   _____ D. Common iliac artery and vein

5. Which of the following is illustrated by 1?
   _____ A. Cecum
   _____ B. Descending colon
   _____ C. Sigmoid colon
   _____ D. Small bowel

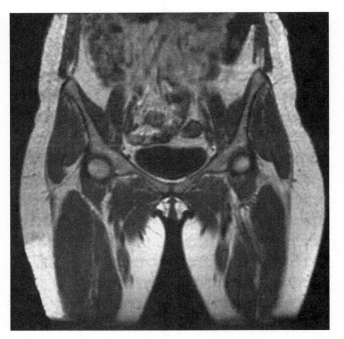

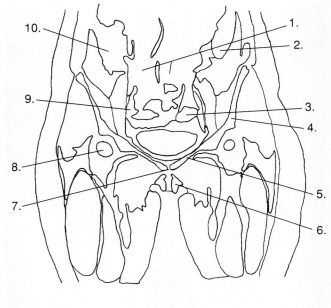

Figure 4-48

1. Which of the following is illustrated by 6?
   _____ A. Labium minora
   _____ B. Pelvic diaphragm
   _____ C. Labium majora
   _____ D. Ischiorectal fossa

2. Which of the following is illustrated by 9?
   _____ A. Internal iliac artery and vein
   _____ B. External iliac artery and vein
   _____ C. Femoral artery and vein
   _____ D. Common iliac artery and vein

3. Which number illustrates the descending colon?
   _____ A. 10
   _____ B. 1
   _____ C. 2
   _____ D. 3

4. Which of the following is illustrated by 5?
   _____ A. Ilium
   _____ B. Ischium
   _____ C. Pubis
   _____ D. Pelvic diaphragm

5. Which number illustrates the sigmoid colon?
   _____ A. 10
   _____ B. 1
   _____ C. 2
   _____ D. 3

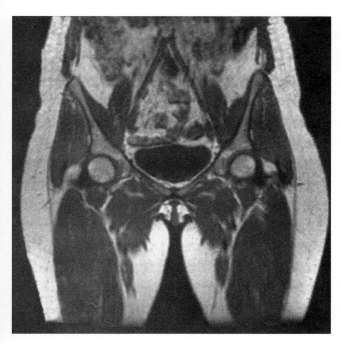
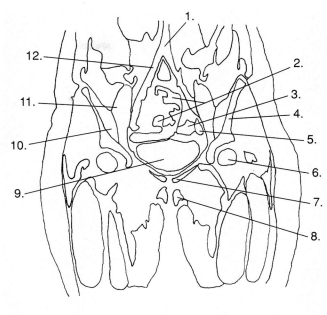

Figure 4-49

1. Which of the following is illustrated by 12?
   _____ A. Internal iliac artery and vein
   _____ B. External iliac artery and vein
   _____ C. Femoral artery and vein
   _____ D. Common iliac artery

2. Which number illustrates the small bowel?
   _____ A. 3
   _____ B. 2
   _____ C. 9
   _____ D. 11

3. Which number illustrates the iliacus muscle?
   _____ A. 5
   _____ B. 4
   _____ C. 11
   _____ D. 10

4. Which of the following is illustrated by 7?
   _____ A. Ilium
   _____ B. Ischium
   _____ C. Pubis
   _____ D. Pelvic diaphragm

5. Which of the following is illustrated by 5?
   _____ A. Internal iliac artery and vein
   _____ B. External iliac artery and vein
   _____ C. Femoral artery and vein
   _____ D. Common iliac artery and vein

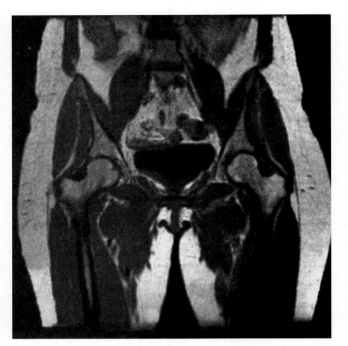

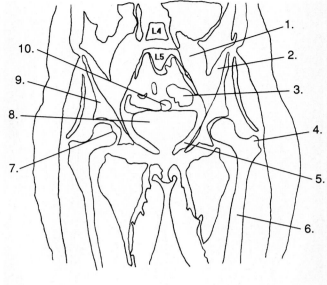

Figure 4-50

1. Which of the following is illustrated by 1?
_____ A. Descending colon
_____ B. Sigmoid colon
_____ C. Psoas muscle
_____ D. Iliacus muscle

2. Which of the following is illustrated by 7?
_____ A. Greater trochanter of femur
_____ B. Shaft of femur
_____ C. Fovea capitis femoris
_____ D. Lesser trochanter of femur

3. Which of the following is illustrated by 10?
_____ A. Small bowel
_____ B. Sigmoid colon
_____ C. Cecum
_____ D. Descending colon

4. Which number illustrates the bladder?
_____ A. 3
_____ B. 10
_____ C. 8
_____ D. 9

5. Which number illustrates the ilium?
_____ A. 3
_____ B. 10
_____ C. 9
_____ D. 8

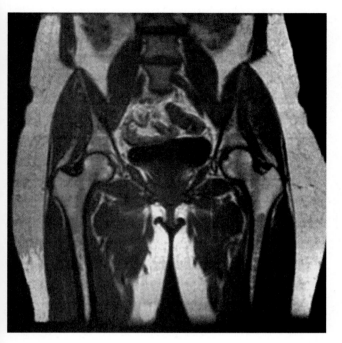

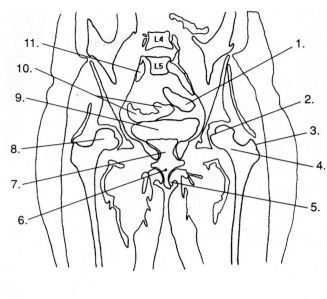

Figure 4-51

1. Which of the following is illustrated by 1?
   _____ A. Small bowel
   _____ B. Sigmoid colon
   _____ C. Psoas muscle
   _____ D. Iliacus muscle

2. Which of the following is illustrated by 11?
   _____ A. Internal iliac artery and vein
   _____ B. External iliac artery and vein
   _____ C. Femoral artery and vein
   _____ D. Common iliac artery and vein

3. Which of the following is illustrated by 7?
   _____ A. Uterus
   _____ B. Wall of bladder
   _____ C. Pelvic diaphragm
   _____ D. Cervix

4. Which of the following is illustrated by 6?
   _____ A. Ureter
   _____ B. Urethra
   _____ C. Vagina
   _____ D. Vaginal fornix

5. Which number illustrates the urethra?
   _____ A. 5
   _____ B. 6
   _____ C. 7
   _____ D. 9

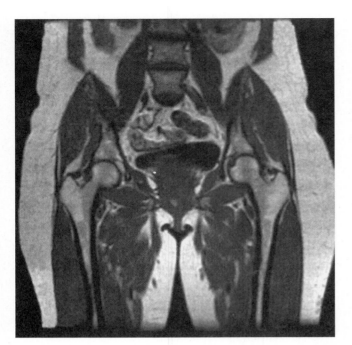

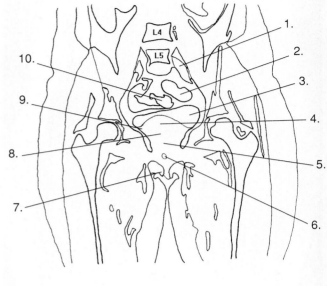

Figure 4-52

1. Which number illustrates the adnexal area?
    _____ A. 4
    _____ B. 5
    _____ C. 8
    _____ D. 9

2. Which number illustrates the cervix?
    _____ A. 4
    _____ B. 8
    _____ C. 5
    _____ D. 6

3. Which of the following is illustrated by 6?
    _____ A. Urethra
    _____ B. Cervix of uterus
    _____ C. Vagina
    _____ D. Rectum

4. Which of the following is illustrated by 3?
    _____ A. Posterior bladder
    _____ B. Sigmoid colon
    _____ C. Small bowel
    _____ D. Body of uterus

5. Which of the following is illustrated by 4?
    _____ A. Adnexal area
    _____ B. Cervix of uterus
    _____ C. Posterior bladder
    _____ D. Fundus of uterus

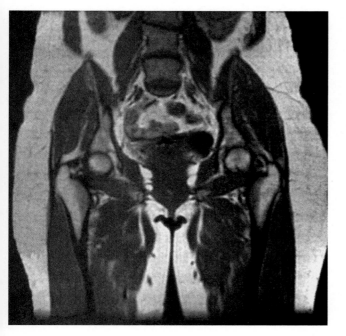

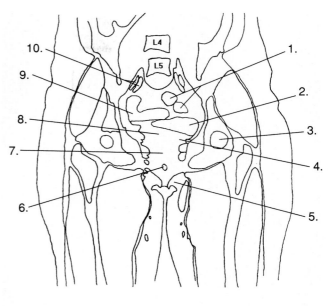

Figure 4-53

1. Which number illustrates the sigmoid colon?
   _____ A. 9
   _____ B. 1
   _____ C. 2
   _____ D. 8

2. Which of the following is illustrated by 7?
   _____ A. Urethra
   _____ B. Cervix of uterus
   _____ C. Vagina
   _____ D. Rectum

3. Which of the following is illustrated by 4?
   _____ A. Adnexal area
   _____ B. Cervix of uterus
   _____ C. Posterior bladder
   _____ D. Fundus of uterus

4. Which of the following is illustrated by 3?
   _____ A. Ischium
   _____ B. Femur
   _____ C. Ilium
   _____ D. Pubis

5. Which of the following is illustrated by 10?
   _____ A. Internal iliac artery and vein
   _____ B. External iliac artery and vein
   _____ C. Common iliac artery and vein
   _____ D. Femoral artery and vein

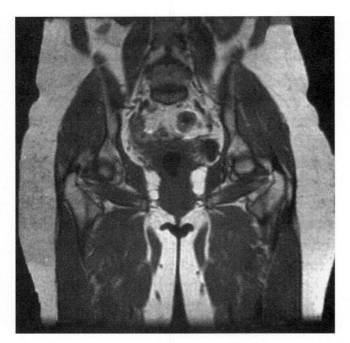

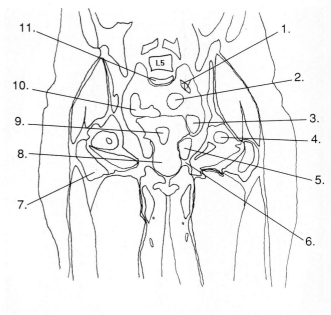

Figure 4-54

1. Which of the following is illustrated by 8?
   _____ A. Vagina
   _____ B. Urethra
   _____ C. Anal sphincter
   _____ D. Ischiorectal fossa

2. Which of the following is illustrated by 9?
   _____ A. Urethra
   _____ B. Vagina
   _____ C. Rectum
   _____ D. Sigmoid colon

3. Which of the following is illustrated by 3?
   _____ A. Small bowel
   _____ B. Sigmoid colon
   _____ C. Adnexal area
   _____ D. Posterior bladder

4. Which number illustrates the pelvic diaphragm?
   _____ A. 6
   _____ B. 8
   _____ C. 5
   _____ D. 7

5. Which of the following is illustrated by 1?
   _____ A. Common iliac artery and vein
   _____ B. Internal iliac artery and vein
   _____ C. External iliac artery and vein
   _____ D. Gluteal artery and vein

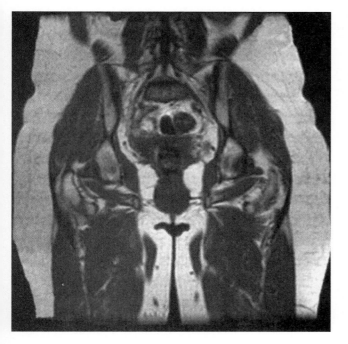
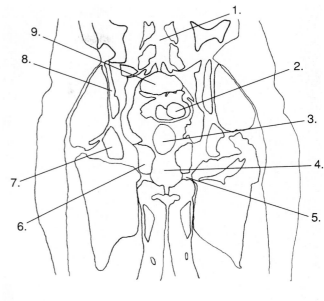

Figure 4-55

1. Which of the following is illustrated by 7?
   _____ A. Ilium
   _____ B. Ischial tuberosity
   _____ C. Pubis
   _____ D. Ischial spine

2. Which of the following is illustrated by 3?
   _____ A. Rectum
   _____ B. Vagina
   _____ C. Sigmoid colon
   _____ D. Small bowel

3. Which number illustrates the vertebral foramen?
   _____ A. 1
   _____ B. 9
   _____ C. 2
   _____ D. 3

4. Which number illustrates the rectum?
   _____ A. 2
   _____ B. 3
   _____ C. 4
   _____ D. 9

5. Which number illustrates the ilium?
   _____ A. 6
   _____ B. 7
   _____ C. 8
   _____ D. 9

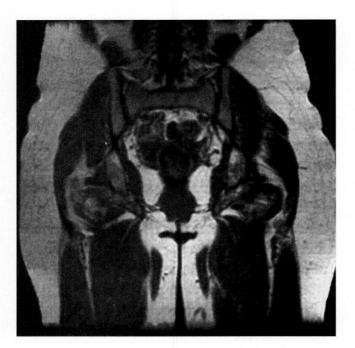
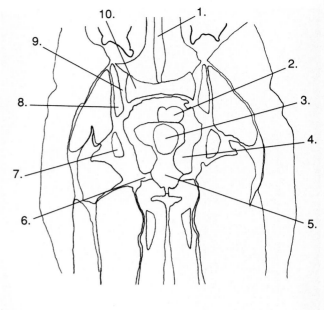

Figure 4-56

1. Which of the following is illustrated by 9?
   _____ A. Ilium
   _____ B. Sacroiliac joint
   _____ C. Sacrum
   _____ D. Ischial tuberosity

2. Which of the following is illustrated by 5?
   _____ A. Rectum
   _____ B. Vagina
   _____ C. Anal sphincter
   _____ D. Pelvic diaphragm

3. Which number illustrates the ischial tuberosity?
   _____ A. 9
   _____ B. 8
   _____ C. 7
   _____ D. 6

4. Which of the following is illustrated by 3?
   _____ A. Rectum
   _____ B. Vagina
   _____ C. Sigmoid colon
   _____ D. Anal sphincter

5. Which number illustrates the sigmoid colon?
   _____ A. 1
   _____ B. 2
   _____ C. 3
   _____ D. 5

CLINICAL APPLICATIONS

----

1. Which of the following is considered retroperitoneal in location?
   - _____ A. Ileum
   - _____ B. Transverse colon
   - _____ C. Jejunum
   - _____ D. Ascending colon

2. Which of the following is the erectile tissue forming the anterior part of the penis?
   - _____ A. Cavernosum spongiosum
   - _____ B. Corpus cavernosum
   - _____ C. Corpus spongiosum
   - _____ D. Cavernosum spongiosum

3. Which of the following structures would be considered most posterior in the pelvis?
   - _____ A. Lower bladder
   - _____ B. Urethra
   - _____ C. Prostate
   - _____ D. Seminal vesicles

4. All of the following muscles form the pelvic diaphragm except the:
   - _____ A. Iliacus
   - _____ B. Levator ani
   - _____ C. Coccygeus
   - _____ D. All of the above from the pelvic diaphragm

5. The femoral artery originates from the:
   - _____ A. Common iliac artery
   - _____ B. Gluteal artery
   - _____ C. External iliac artery
   - _____ D. Internal iliac artery

6. In an axial section through the pelvis, which alimentary structure would be most inferior?
   - _____ A. Ascending colon
   - _____ B. Descending colon
   - _____ C. Sigmoid colon
   - _____ D. Rectum

7. Which of the following is located most inferiorly?
   - _____ A. Acetabulum
   - _____ B. Coccyx
   - _____ C. Symphysis pubis
   - _____ D. Obturator foramen

8. Which of the following best describes the position of the greater trochanter of the femur?
   - _____ A. Anterior and medial
   - _____ B. Posterior and medial
   - _____ C. Anterior and lateral
   - _____ D. Posterior and lateral

9. The most distinctive difference between the lower segments of the sacrum and the coccyx is the absence of the _____.

10. What space surrounds the cervix of the uterus extending into the vagina?

    _____

    _____

    _____

CLINICAL CORRELATIONS

■ Clinical Case 4-1

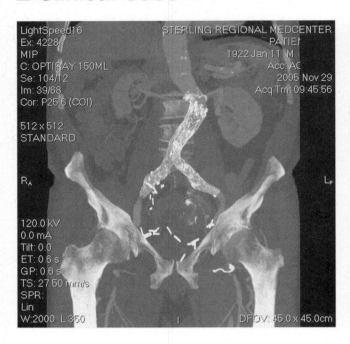 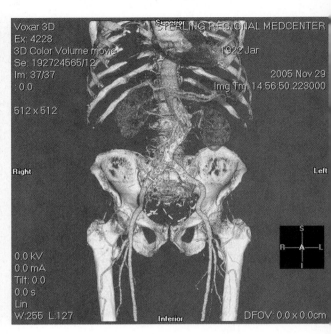

1. Both images provided above were generated during which of the following procedures?
   _____ A. Computed tomography angiography (CTA)
   _____ B. Magnetic resonance angiography (MRA)
   _____ C. Ultrasound
   _____ D. Positron emission tomography/computed tomography (PET/CT)

2. In this patient, the stent graft has been placed in which of the following?
   _____ A. Right common iliac artery
   _____ B. Left common iliac artery
   _____ C. Abdominal aorta
   _____ D. All of the above

3. Which of the following best describes how the internal iliac arteries exit the pelvis?
   _____ A. Obturator foramina
   _____ B. Posterior bony pelvis
   _____ C. Sacral foramina
   _____ D. Anterior bony pelvis

4. Does the endograft appear to be patent?
   _____ A. Yes
   _____ B. No

5. The external iliac artery gives rise to the femoral artery after passing which of the following anatomic landmarks?
   _____ A. Sacral promontory
   _____ B. Greater sciatic notch
   _____ C. Ilium
   _____ D. Pubic bone

■ Clinical Case 4-2

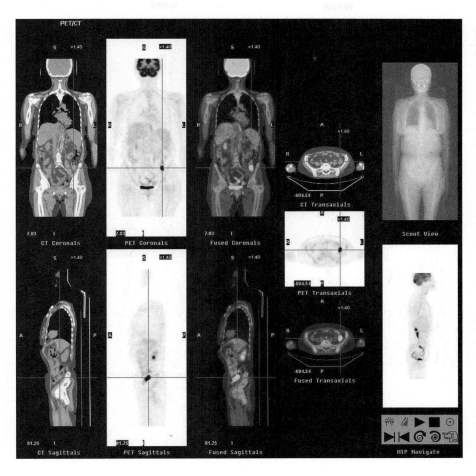

1. According to the marker lines, increased metabolic rate was detected in which of the following?
   _____ A. Cecum
   _____ B. Sigmoid
   _____ C. Ascending colon
   _____ D. Descending colon

2. The strong signal demonstrated in the midline of the pelvis would best be described by which of the following?
   _____ A. Prostate
   _____ B. Uterus
   _____ C. Urinary bladder
   _____ D. Seminal vesicles

3. Which of the following is the lower part of the large bowel found in the right greater pelvis?
   _____ A. Cecum
   _____ B. Sigmoid colon
   _____ C. Ascending colon
   _____ D. Descending colon

4. On the CT image, which part of the bowel would most likely be sectioned in the anterior part of the greater pelvis?
   _____ A. Cecum
   _____ B. Sigmoid colon
   _____ C. Ileum
   _____ D. Jejunum

5. In a sequence of axial sections, which of the following would be the most inferior part of the large bowel?
   _____ A. Cecum
   _____ B. Sigmoid colon
   _____ C. Ascending colon
   _____ D. Descending colon

■ Clinical Case 4-3

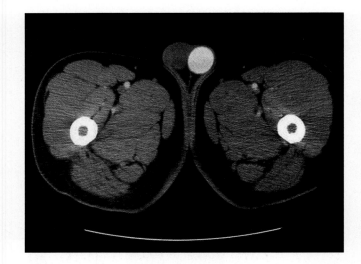

1. In this axial CT image, describe the location of the testicular prosthesis in this young male patient previously treated for testicular seminoma.

    _____

    _____

    _____

2. Describe the changes in adjacent tissues.

    _____

    _____

    _____

3. Describe the consistency, shape, and border.

    _____

    _____

    _____

Clinical Case 4-4

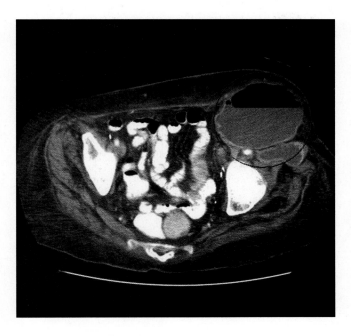

1. Describe the location of the pelvic abscess originating from an infected diverticulum in the descending colon as shown in this axial CT image through the lower abdomen.

   _____

   _____

   _____

2. Describe the changes in adjacent tissues.

   _____

   _____

   _____

3. Describe the consistency, shape, and border.

   _____

   _____

   _____

■ Clinical Case 4-5

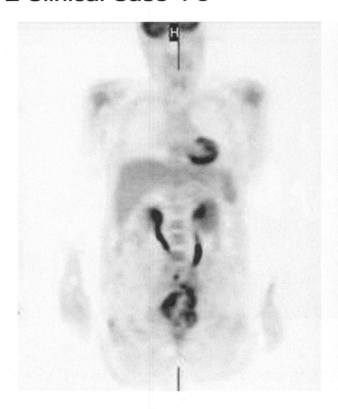 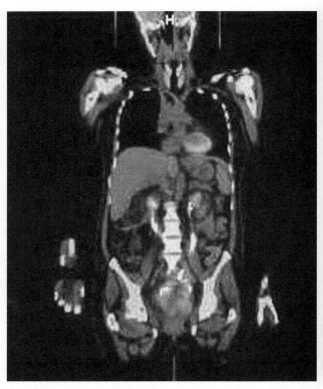

1. Describe the location of the adenocarcinoma shown in this 47-year-old female. The PET image is shown on the left with a corresponding fused PET/CT image on the right.

   _____

   _____

   _____

2. Describe the changes in adjacent tissues.

   _____

   _____

   _____

3. Describe the consistency, shape, and border.

   _____

   _____

   _____

■ Clinical Case 4-6

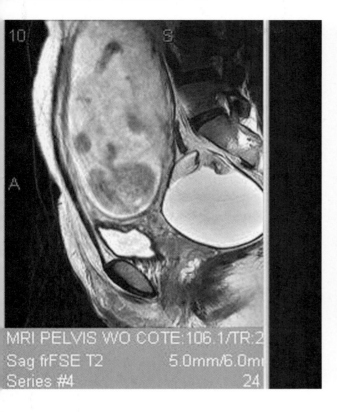
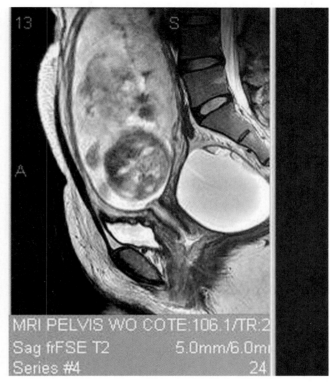

1. Describe the location of the cystic mass found on the selected MR saggital images of this pregnant patient.

   _____

   _____

   _____

2. Describe the changes in adjacent tissues.

   _____

   _____

   _____

3. Describe the consistency, shape, and border.

   _____

   _____

   _____

■ Clinical Case 4-7

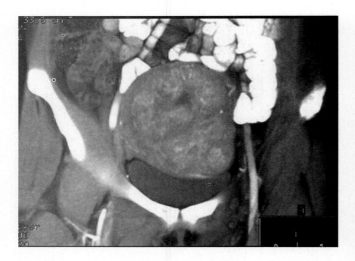 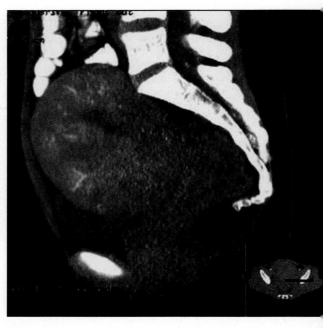

1. Describe the location of the uterine fibroid shown in the coronal (left) and saggital (right) CT images.

   _____

   _____

   _____

2. Describe the changes in adjacent tissues.

   _____

   _____

   _____

3. Describe the consistency, shape, and border.

   _____

   _____

   _____

■ Clinical Case 4-8

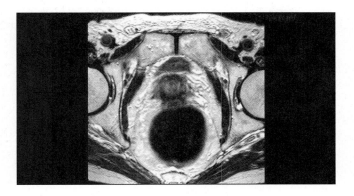

1. Describe the location of the prostate carcinoma in the axial MR section of this 81-year-old male patient.

_____

_____

_____

2. Describe the changes in adjacent tissues.

_____

_____

_____

3. Describe the consistency, shape, and border.

_____

_____

_____

Head

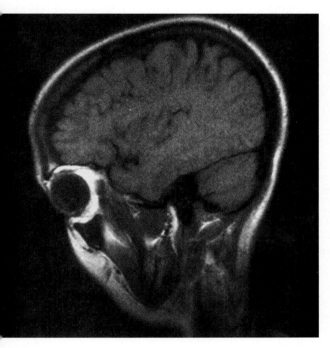
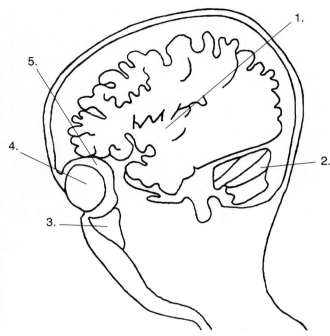

Figure 5-1

1. Which number illustrates the insula?
   _____ A. 5
   _____ B. 2
   _____ C. 1
   _____ D. 3

2. Which of the following is illustrated by 3?
   _____ A. Maxillary sinus
   _____ B. Sphenoid sinus
   _____ C. Frontal sinus
   _____ D. Mastoid air cells

3. Which number illustrates the cerebellum?
   _____ A. 3
   _____ B. 5
   _____ C. 2
   _____ D. 1

4. Which of the following is illustrated by 5?
   _____ A. Sulci
   _____ B. Inferior rectus muscle
   _____ C. Fat in bony orbit
   _____ D. Maxillary sinus

5. Which of the following is illustrated by 4?
   _____ A. Globe of the eye
   _____ B. Superior rectus muscle
   _____ C. Optic nerve
   _____ D. Inferior rectus muscle

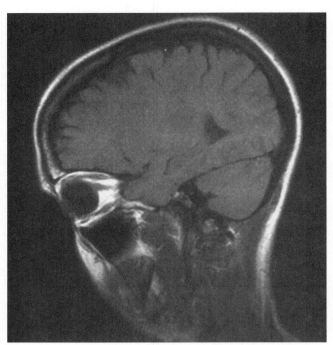
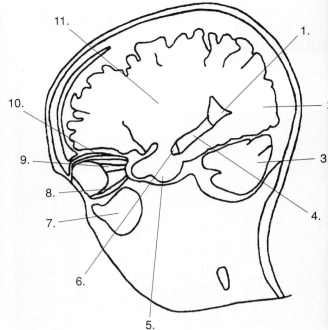

Figure 5-2

1. Which of the following is illustrated by 4?
   _____ A. Posterior horn of the lateral ventricle
   _____ B. Body of caudate nucleus
   _____ C. Thalamus
   _____ D. Inferior horn of the lateral ventricle

2. Which number illustrates the inferior horn of the lateral ventricle?
   _____ A. 6
   _____ B. 4
   _____ C. 1
   _____ D. 7

3. Which of the following is illustrated by 1?
   _____ A. Body of caudate nucleus
   _____ B. Insula
   _____ C. Posterior horn of the lateral ventricle
   _____ D. Inferior horn of the lateral ventricle

4. Which of the following is illustrated by 9?
   _____ A. Superior rectus muscle
   _____ B. Inferior rectus muscle
   _____ C. Optic nerve
   _____ D. Fat in bony orbit

5. Which number illustrates the superior rectus muscle?
   _____ A. 9
   _____ B. 6
   _____ C. 8
   _____ D. 10

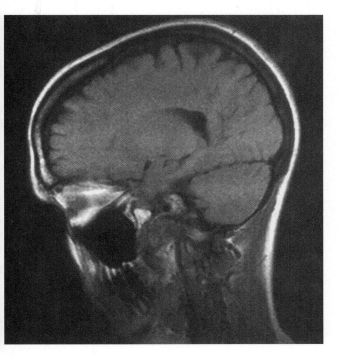

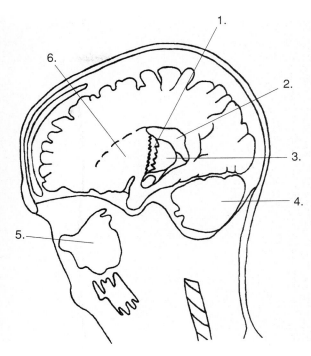

Figure 5-3

1. Which of the following is illustrated by 6?
  _____ A. Thalamus
  _____ B. Lenticular nuclei
  _____ C. Insula
  _____ D. Occipital lobe

2. Which number illustrates the internal capsule?
  _____ A. 3
  _____ B. 2
  _____ C. 6
  _____ D. 1

3. Which of the following is illustrated by 5?
  _____ A. Maxillary sinus
  _____ B. Frontal sinus
  _____ C. Fat in bony orbit
  _____ D. Insula

4. Which number illustrates the cerebellum?
  _____ A. 3
  _____ B. 4
  _____ C. 5
  _____ D. 2

5. Which of the following is illustrated by 3?
  _____ A. Lenticular nuclei
  _____ B. Body of caudate nucleus
  _____ C. Thalamus
  _____ D. Internal capsule

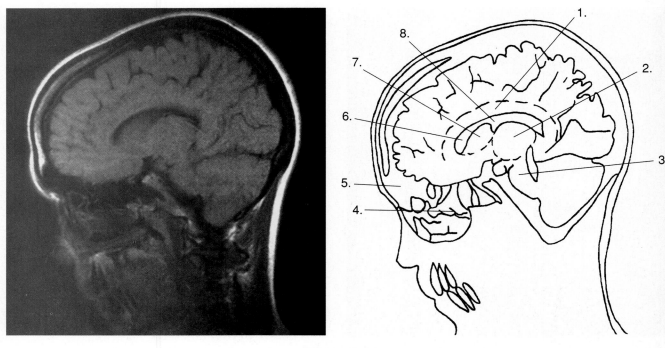

Figure 5-4

1. Which of the following is illustrated by 8?
   _____ A. Thalamus
   _____ B. Body of lateral ventricle
   _____ C. Head of caudate
   _____ D. Corpus callosum

2. Which number illustrates the anterior horn of the lateral ventricle?
   _____ A. 8
   _____ B. 2
   _____ C. 7
   _____ D. 6

3. Which of the following is illustrated by 5?
   _____ A. Maxillary sinus
   _____ B. Ethmoid sinus
   _____ C. Frontal sinus
   _____ D. Fat in bony orbit

4. Which number illustrates the corpus callosum?
   _____ A. 1
   _____ B. 8
   _____ C. 7
   _____ D. 6

5. Which of the following is illustrated by 7?
   _____ A. Thalamus
   _____ B. Head of caudate
   _____ C. Intermediate mass
   _____ D. Body of lateral ventricle

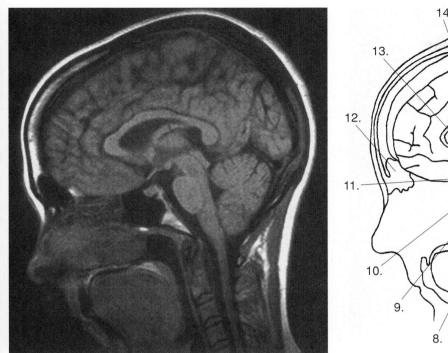

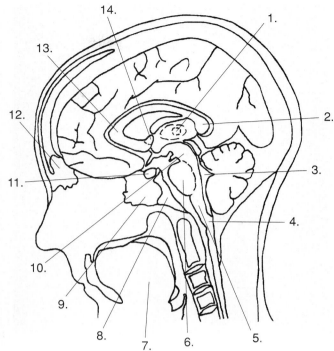

Figure 5-5

1. Which number illustrates the splenium of corpus callosum?
   _____ A. 1
   _____ B. 13
   _____ C. 2
   _____ D. 14

2. Which of the following is illustrated by 10?
   _____ A. Pons
   _____ B. Cerebral peduncles
   _____ C. Pituitary gland
   _____ D. Quadrigeminal plate

3. Which number illustrates the pituitary gland?
   _____ A. 11
   _____ B. 3
   _____ C. 10
   _____ D. 6

4. Which of the following is illustrated by 1?
   _____ A. Head of caudate nucleus
   _____ B. Anterior commissure
   _____ C. Intermediate mass
   _____ D. Splenium of corpus callosum

5. Which of the following is illustrated by 14?
   _____ A. Intermediate mass
   _____ B. Pituitary gland
   _____ C. Genu of corpus callosum
   _____ D. Anterior commissure

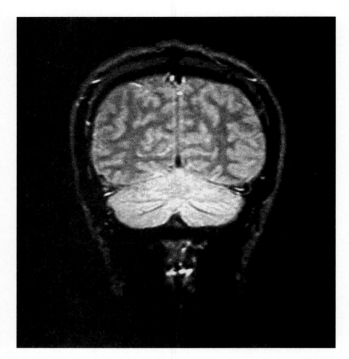

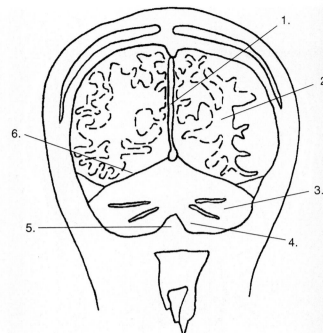

Figure 5-6

1. Which of the following is demonstrated by 2?
   _____ A. Occipital lobe
   _____ B. Parietal lobe
   _____ C. Cerebellar hemisphere
   _____ D. Temporal lobe

2. Which number illustrates the cisterna magna?
   _____ A. 6
   _____ B. 1
   _____ C. 5
   _____ D. 4

3. Which of the following is demonstrated by 1?
   _____ A. Straight sinus
   _____ B. Falx cerebri
   _____ C. Superior sagittal sinus
   _____ D. Falx cerebelli

4. Which number illustrates the cerebellar tonsil?
   _____ A. 3
   _____ B. 5
   _____ C. 6
   _____ D. 4

5. Which of the following is demonstrated by 3?
   _____ A. Cerebellar hemisphere
   _____ B. Cerebellar tonsil
   _____ C. Occipital lobe
   _____ D. Temporal lobe

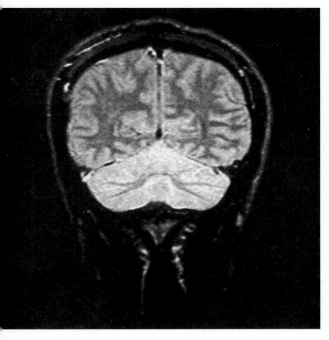
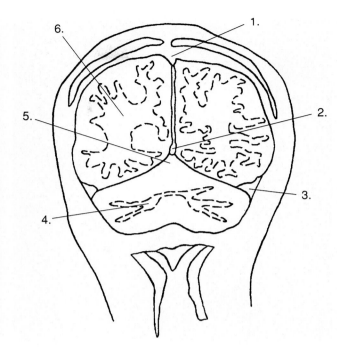

Figure 5-7

1. Which number illustrates the occipital lobe white matter?
   _____ A. 3
   _____ B. 1
   _____ C. 6
   _____ D. 4

2. Which of the following is illustrated by 1?
   _____ A. Straight sinus
   _____ B. Superior sagittal sinus
   _____ C. Transverse sinus
   _____ D. Cisterna magna

3. Which number illustrates the superior cerebellar vermis?
   _____ A. 5
   _____ B. 1
   _____ C. 3
   _____ D. 2

4. Which of the following is illustrated by 2?
   _____ A. Straight sinus
   _____ B. Superior sagittal sinus
   _____ C. Transverse sinus
   _____ D. Cisterna magna

5. Which of the following is illustrated by 3?
   _____ A. Superior sagittal sinus
   _____ B. Cisterna magna
   _____ C. Straight sinus
   _____ D. Transverse sinus

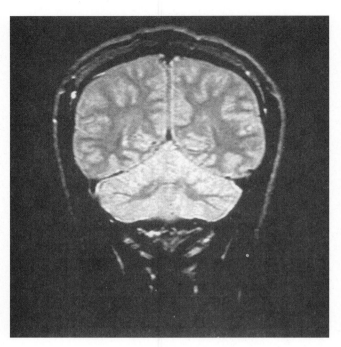
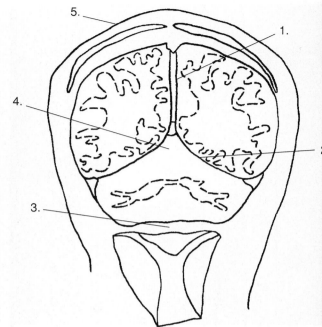

Figure 5-8

1. Which of the following is illustrated by 5?
   _____ A. Parietal bone
   _____ B. Scalp
   _____ C. Tentorium cerebelli
   _____ D. Occipital bone

2. Which number illustrates the superior cerebellar vermis?
   _____ A. 4
   _____ B. 2
   _____ C. 3
   _____ D. 1

3. Which of the following is illustrated by 1?
   _____ A. Straight sinus
   _____ B. Superior sagittal sinus
   _____ C. Falx cerebri
   _____ D. Falx cerebelli

4. Which number illustrates the tentorium cerebelli?
   _____ A. 3
   _____ B. 1
   _____ C. 4
   _____ D. 2

5. Which of the following is illustrated by 3?
   _____ A. Scalp
   _____ B. Occipital bone
   _____ C. Posterior medulla oblongata
   _____ D. Cisterna magna

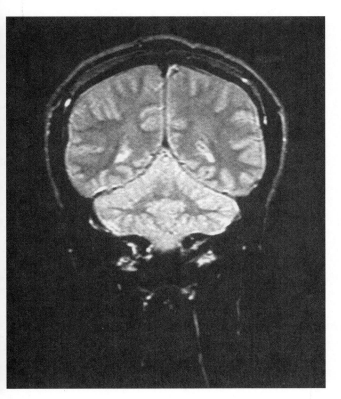 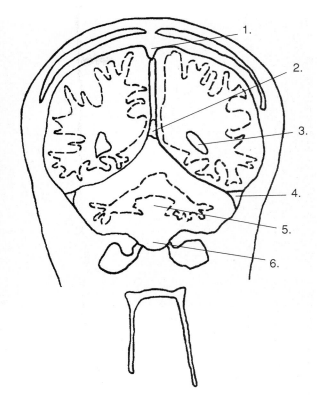

Figure 5-9

1. Which number illustrates the fourth ventricle?
   _____ A. 3
   _____ B. 1
   _____ C. 5
   _____ D. 6

2. Which of the following is illustrated by 1?
   _____ A. Straight sinus
   _____ B. Superior sagittal sinus
   _____ C. Cisterna magna
   _____ D. Fourth ventricle

3. Which of the following is illustrated by 4?
   _____ A. Superior sagittal sinus
   _____ B. Transverse sinus
   _____ C. Straight sinus
   _____ D. Confluence of sinuses

4. Which number illustrates the straight sinus?
   _____ A. 4
   _____ B. 5
   _____ C. 1
   _____ D. 2

5. Which of the following is illustrated by 3?
   _____ A. Posterior horn of the lateral ventricle
   _____ B. Anterior horn of the lateral ventricle
   _____ C. Cisterna magna
   _____ D. Fourth ventricle

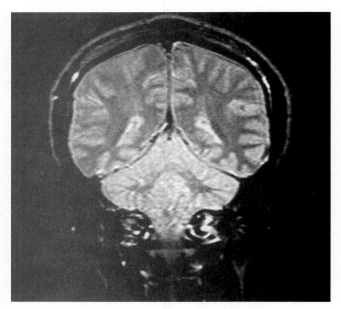
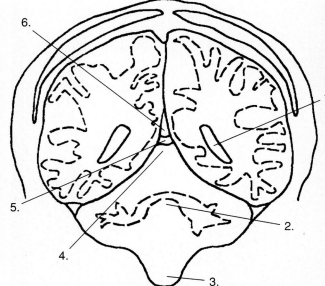

Figure 5-10

1. Which number illustrates the fourth ventricle?
   _____ A. 6
   _____ B. 1
   _____ C. 5
   _____ D. 2

2. Which of the following is illustrated by 6?
   _____ A. Superior sagittal sinus
   _____ B. Straight sinus
   _____ C. Transverse sinus
   _____ D. Fourth ventricle

3. Which number illustrates the superior cerebellar vermis?
   _____ A. 4
   _____ B. 6
   _____ C. 1
   _____ D. 5

4. Which of the following is illustrated by 5?
   _____ A. Superior cerebellar vermis
   _____ B. Straight sinus
   _____ C. Superior cistern
   _____ D. Fourth ventricle

5. Which of the following is illustrated by 1?
   _____ A. Posterior horn of the lateral ventricle
   _____ B. Transverse sinus
   _____ C. Straight sinus
   _____ D. Fourth ventricle

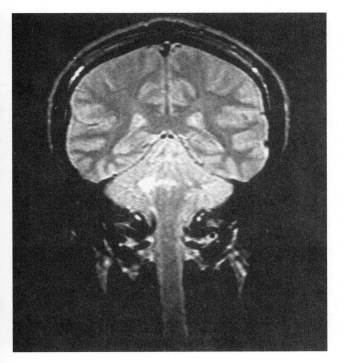
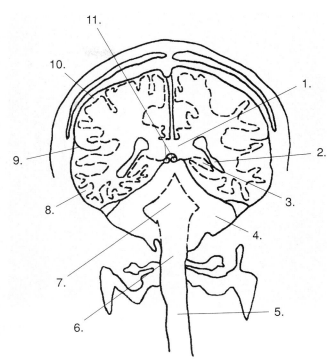

Figure 5-11

1. Which number illustrates the posterior pons?
   _____ A. 11
   _____ B. 6
   _____ C. 5
   _____ D. 7

2. Which of the following is illustrated by 1?
   _____ A. Splenium of corpus callosum
   _____ B. Hippocampal formation
   _____ C. Anterior commissure
   _____ D. Genu of corpus callosum

3. Which of the following is illustrated by 9?
   _____ A. Sylvian fissure
   _____ B. Collateral trigone of the lateral ventricle
   _____ C. Splenium of corpus callosum
   _____ D. Superior cistern

4. Which number illustrates the hippocampal formation?
   _____ A. 2
   _____ B. 1
   _____ C. 3
   _____ D. 11

5. Which number illustrates the collateral trigone of the lateral ventricle?
   _____ A. 2
   _____ B. 9
   _____ C. 3
   _____ D. 1

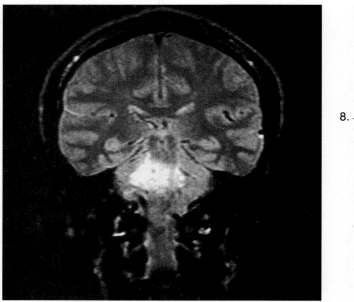
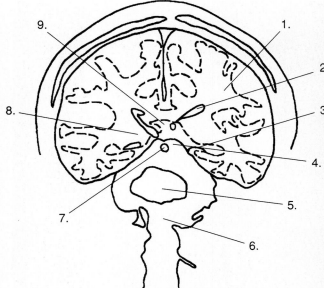

Figure 5-12

1. Which of the following is illustrated by 4?
   _____ A. Quadrigeminal plate
   _____ B. Cerebral aqueduct
   _____ C. Medulla oblongata
   _____ D. Corona radiata

2. Which number illustrates the pineal gland?
   _____ A. 7
   _____ B. 9
   _____ C. 3
   _____ D. 2

3. Which number illustrates the cerebral aqueduct?
   _____ A. 5
   _____ B. 4
   _____ C. 7
   _____ D. 9

4. Which of the following is illustrated by 1?
   _____ A. Quadrigeminal plate
   _____ B. Corona radiata
   _____ C. Thalamus
   _____ D. Body of lateral ventricle

5. Which number illustrates the inferior horn of the lateral ventricle?
   _____ A. 7
   _____ B. 9
   _____ C. 2
   _____ D. 3

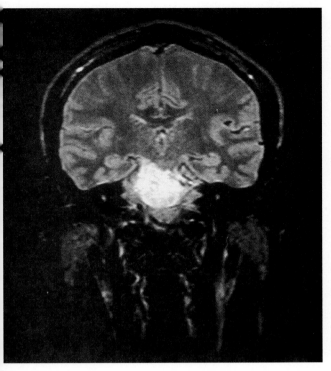
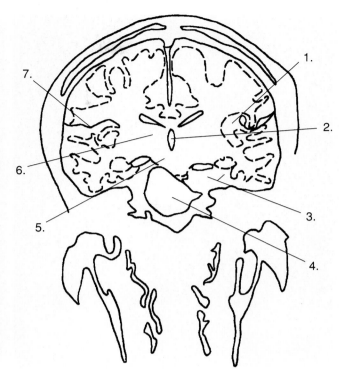

Figure 5-13

1. Which of the following is illustrated by 3?
   _____ A. Hippocampal formation
   _____ B. Sylvian fissure
   _____ C. Head of caudate nucleus
   _____ D. Quadrigeminal plate

2. Which number illustrates the insula?
   _____ A. 6
   _____ B. 5
   _____ C. 7
   _____ D. 1

3. Which of the following is illustrated by 2?
   _____ A. Pineal gland
   _____ B. Third ventricle
   _____ C. Pons
   _____ D. Cerebral aqueduct

4. Which of the following is illustrated by 6?
   _____ A. Sylvian fissure
   _____ B. Thalamus
   _____ C. Insula
   _____ D. Lenticular nuclei

5. Which number illustrates the cerebral peduncles?
   _____ A. 3
   _____ B. 6
   _____ C. 1
   _____ D. 5

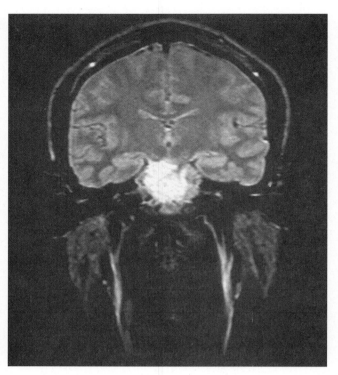

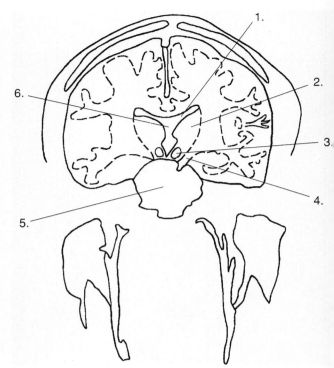

Figure 5-14

1. Which number illustrates the thalamus?
   _____ A. 1
   _____ B. 3
   _____ C. 6
   _____ D. 2

2. Which of the following is illustrated by 4?
   _____ A. Red nucleus
   _____ B. Substantia nigra
   _____ C. Quadrigeminal formation
   _____ D. Quadrigeminal plate

3. Which number illustrates the red nucleus?
   _____ A. 3
   _____ B. 6
   _____ C. 4
   _____ D. 1

4. Which of the following is illustrated by 1?
   _____ A. Insula
   _____ B. Thalamus
   _____ C. Third ventricle
   _____ D. Body of lateral ventricle

5. Which of the following is illustrated by 6?
   _____ A. Fourth ventricle
   _____ B. Collateral trigone of lateral ventricle
   _____ C. Third ventricle
   _____ D. Body of lateral ventricle

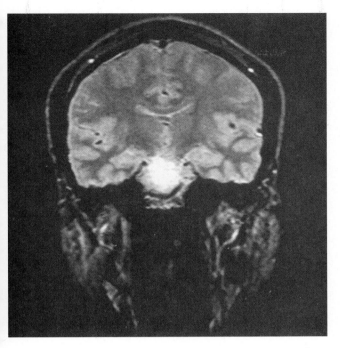

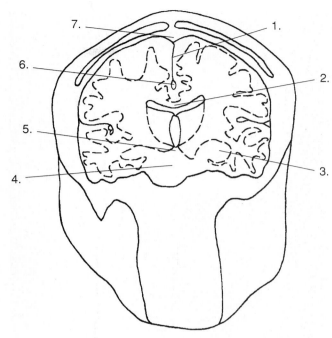

Figure 5-15

1. Which number illustrates the body of corpus callosum?
   _____ A. 2
   _____ B. 1
   _____ C. 3
   _____ D. 1

2. Which of the following is illustrated by 4?
   _____ A. Hippocampal formation
   _____ B. Quadrigeminal plate
   _____ C. Midbrain
   _____ D. Pons

3. Which of the following is illustrated by 7?
   _____ A. Superior sagittal sinus
   _____ B. Falx cerebri
   _____ C. Cisterna magna
   _____ D. Inferior sagittal sinus

4. Which number illustrates the midbrain?
   _____ A. 2
   _____ B. 1
   _____ C. 5
   _____ D. 4

5. Which of the following is illustrated by 6?
   _____ A. Superior sagittal sinus
   _____ B. Interior sagittal sinus
   _____ C. Straight sinus
   _____ D. Superior cistern

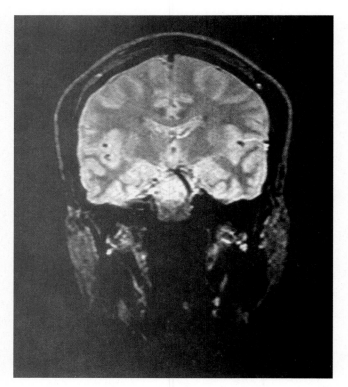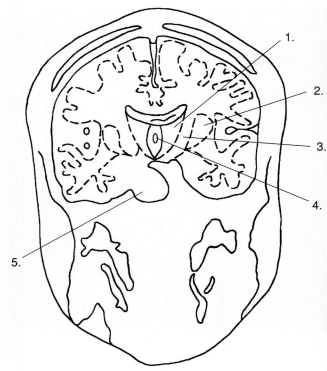

Figure 5-16

1. Which of the following is illustrated by 3?
   _____ A. Thalamus
   _____ B. Body of corpus callosum
   _____ C. Internal capsule
   _____ D. Lenticular nuclei

2. Which of the following is illustrated by 5?
   _____ A. Globus pallidus
   _____ B. Hippocampal formation
   _____ C. Midbrain
   _____ D. Anterior pons

3. Which of the following is illustrated by 2?
   _____ A. Lenticular nuclei
   _____ B. Body of corpus callosum
   _____ C. Internal capsule
   _____ D. Thalamus

4. Which of the following is illustrated by 4?
   _____ A. Superior cistern
   _____ B. Fourth ventricle
   _____ C. Cerebral aqueduct
   _____ D. Third ventricle

5. Which number illustrates the thalamus?
   _____ A. 3
   _____ B. 1
   _____ C. 2
   _____ D. 4

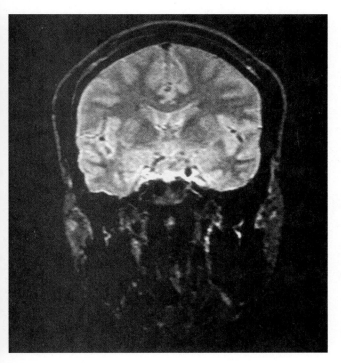
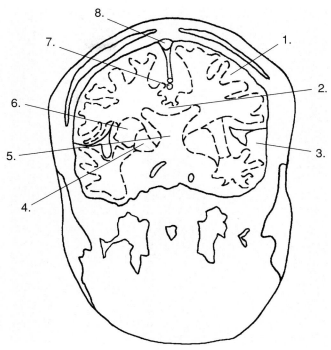

Figure 5-17

1. Which number illustrates the thalamus?
   _____ A. 6
   _____ B. 4
   _____ C. 5
   _____ D. 7

2. Which of the following is illustrated by 1?
   _____ A. Superior sagittal sinus
   _____ B. Parietal lobe
   _____ C. Temporal lobe
   _____ D. Occipital lobe

3. Which of the following is illustrated by 6?
   _____ A. Body of corpus callosum
   _____ B. Globus pallidus
   _____ C. Thalamus
   _____ D. Putamen

4. Which number illustrates the globus pallidus?
   _____ A. 4
   _____ B. 2
   _____ C. 6
   _____ D. 3

5. Which of the following is illustrated by 3?
   _____ A. Occipital lobe
   _____ B. Parietal lobe
   _____ C. Temporal lobe
   _____ D. Globus pallidus

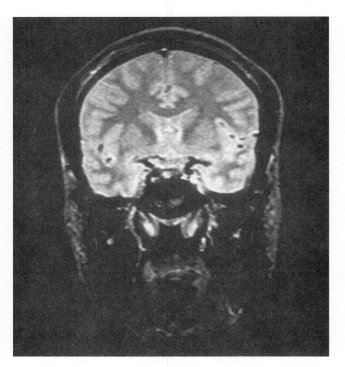
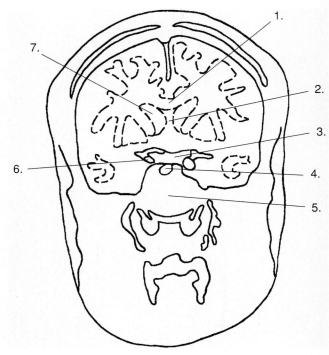

Figure 5-18

1. Which number illustrates the anterior horn of the lateral ventricle?
   _____ A. 7
   _____ B. 2
   _____ C. 1
   _____ D. 5

2. Which of the following is illustrated by 7?
   _____ A. Anterior horn of the lateral ventricle
   _____ B. Body of corpus callosum
   _____ C. Head of the caudate nucleus
   _____ D. Thalamus

3. Which number illustrates the optic chiasma?
   _____ A. 4
   _____ B. 6
   _____ C. 5
   _____ D. 3

4. Which of the following is illustrated by 4?
   _____ A. Pituitary gland
   _____ B. Sphenoid sinus
   _____ C. Third ventricle
   _____ D. Optic chiasma

5. Which of the following is illustrated by 6?
   _____ A. Optic nerve
   _____ B. Pituitary gland
   _____ C. Internal carotid artery
   _____ D. Vertebral artery

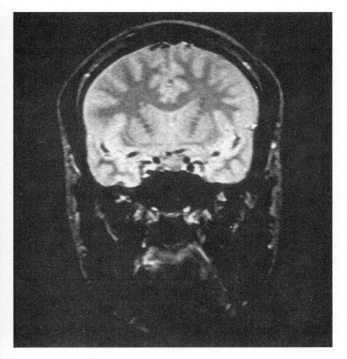 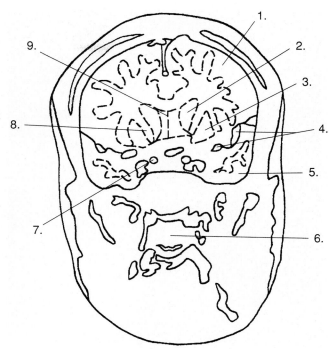

Figure 5-19

1. Which of the following is illustrated by 8?
   _____ A. Internal capsule
   _____ B. Head of caudate nucleus
   _____ C. Globus pallidus
   _____ D. Septum pellucidum

2. Which of the following is illustrated by 3?
   _____ A. Head of caudate nucleus
   _____ B. Septum pellucidum
   _____ C. Lenticular nuclei
   _____ D. Internal carotid artery

3. Which number illustrates the septum pellucidum?
   _____ A. 8
   _____ B. 3
   _____ C. 2
   _____ D. 9

4. Which number illustrates the internal carotid artery?
   _____ A. 7
   _____ B. 3
   _____ C. 2
   _____ D. 4

5. Which of the following is illustrated by 6?
   _____ A. Sphenoid sinus
   _____ B. Nasopharynx
   _____ C. Mastoid sinus
   _____ D. Oropharynx

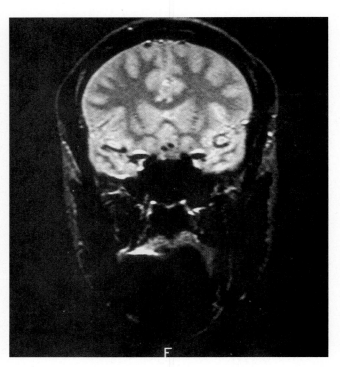
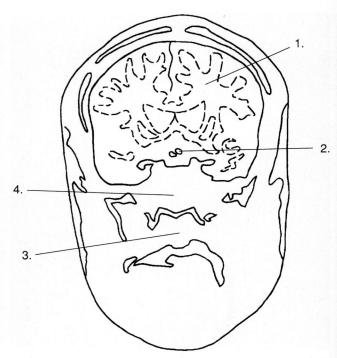

Figure 5-20

1. Which of the following is illustrated by 1?
   _____ A. White matter of parietal lobe
   _____ B. White matter of frontal lobe
   _____ C. Internal capsule
   _____ D. External capsule

2. Which of the following is illustrated by 2?
   _____ A. Straight sinus
   _____ B. Inferior sagittal sinus
   _____ C. Anterior cerebral artery
   _____ D. Middle cerebral artery

3. Which of the following is illustrated by 4?
   _____ A. Sphenoid sinus
   _____ B. Ethmoid air cells
   _____ C. Nasopharynx
   _____ D. Oropharynx

4. Which number illustrates the nasopharynx?
   _____ A. 4
   _____ B. 3
   _____ C. 2
   _____ D. 1

5. Which of the following is illustrated by 3?
   _____ A. Sphenoid sinus
   _____ B. Nasopharynx
   _____ C. Oropharynx
   _____ D. Ethmoid air cells

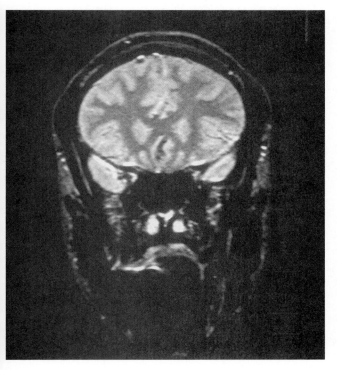

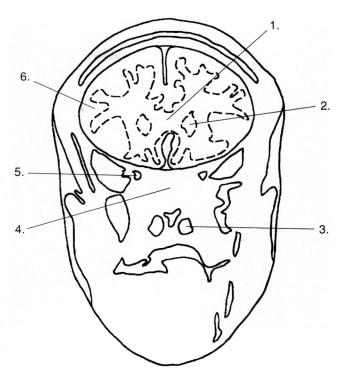

Figure 5-21

1. Which of the following is illustrated by 2?
_____ A. Tail of caudate nucleus
_____ B. Head of caudate nucleus
_____ C. Lenticular nuclei
_____ D. Thalamus

2. Which number illustrates the inferior nasal concha?
_____ A. 5
_____ B. 2
_____ C. 4
_____ D. 3

3. Which of the following is illustrated by 4?
_____ A. Sphenoid sinus
_____ B. Nasopharynx
_____ C. Maxillary sinus
_____ D. Oropharynx

4. Which of the following is illustrated by 1?
_____ A. Head of caudate nucleus
_____ B. Genu of corpus callosum
_____ C. Lenticular nuclei
_____ D. Septum pellucidum

5. Which of the following is illustrated by 5?
_____ A. Anterior cerebral artery
_____ B. Internal carotid artery
_____ C. Optic nerve
_____ D. Posterior cerebral artery

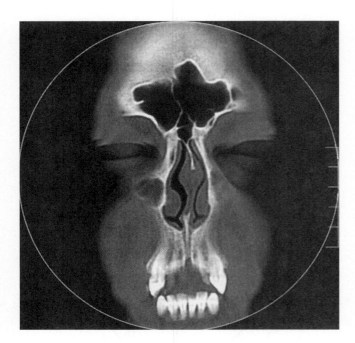

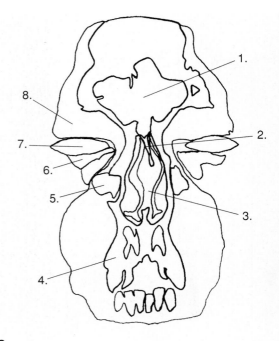

Figure 5-22

1. Which of the following is illustrated by 3?
   _____ A. Septal cartilage
   _____ B. Vomer
   _____ C. Perpendicular plate of ethmoid
   _____ D. Inferior concha

2. Which of the following is illustrated by 5?
   _____ A. Sphenoid sinus
   _____ B. Ethmoid sinus
   _____ C. Maxillary sinus
   _____ D. Frontal sinus

3. Which number illustrates the perpendicular plate of ethmoid?
   _____ A. 3
   _____ B. 2
   _____ C. 4
   _____ D. 1

4. Which number illustrates the frontal sinus?
   _____ A. 5
   _____ B. 3
   _____ C. 4
   _____ D. 1

5. Which number illustrates the maxilla?
   _____ A. 4
   _____ B. 8
   _____ C. 2
   _____ D. 1

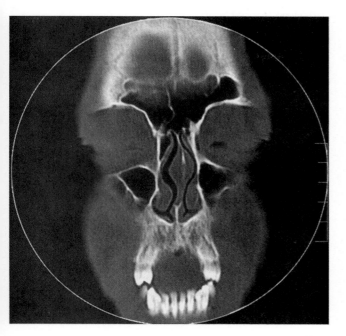

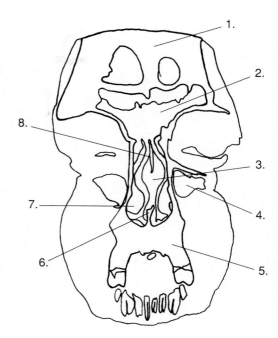

Figure 5-23

1. Which of the following is illustrated by 8?
   _____ A. Septal cartilage
   _____ B. Vomer
   _____ C. Perpendicular plate of ethmoid
   _____ D. Inferior concha

2. Which of the following is illustrated by 6?
   _____ A. Septal cartilage
   _____ B. Vomer
   _____ C. Perpendicular plate of ethmoid
   _____ D. Inferior concha

3. Which number illustrates the inferior concha?
   _____ A. 7
   _____ B. 8
   _____ C. 6
   _____ D. 3

4. Which number illustrates the septal cartilage?
   _____ A. 7
   _____ B. 8
   _____ C. 6
   _____ D. 3

5. Which of the following is illustrated by 5?
   _____ A. Palatine bone
   _____ B. Sphenoid bone
   _____ C. Maxilla bone
   _____ D. Ethmoid bone

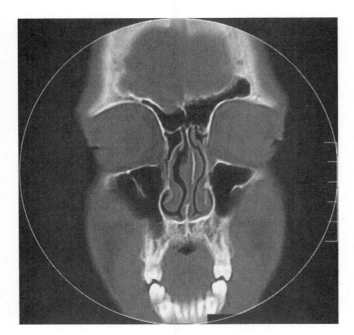
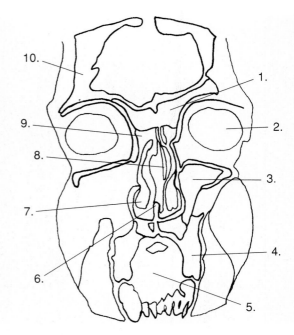

Figure 5-24

1. Which of the following is illustrated by 9?
   _____ A. Sphenoid sinus
   _____ B. Ethmoid sinus
   _____ C. Frontal sinus
   _____ D. Maxillary sinus

2. Which of the following is illustrated by 1?
   _____ A. Sphenoid sinus
   _____ B. Ethmoid sinus
   _____ C. Frontal sinus
   _____ D. Maxillary sinus

3. Which of the following is illustrated by 7?
   _____ A. Inferior concha
   _____ B. Middle concha
   _____ C. Vomer
   _____ D. Septal cartilage

4. Which number illustrates the ethmoid sinus?
   _____ A. 1
   _____ B. 3
   _____ C. 9
   _____ D. 4

5. Which number illustrates the maxillary sinus?
   _____ A. 1
   _____ B. 3
   _____ C. 9
   _____ D. 4

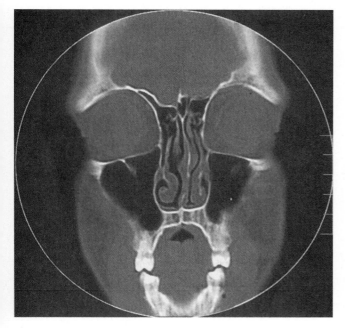

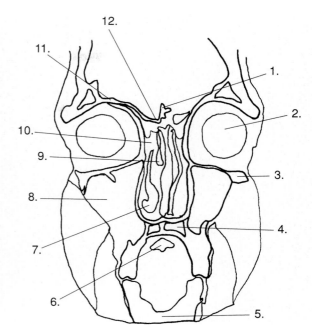

Figure 5-25

1. Which of the following is illustrated by 9?
   _____ A. Superior concha
   _____ B. Middle concha
   _____ C. Inferior concha
   _____ D. Ethmoid sinus

2. Which of the following is illustrated by 1?
   _____ A. Crista galli
   _____ B. Perpendicular plate of ethmoid
   _____ C. Vomer
   _____ D. Cribriform plate

3. Which of the following is illustrated by 12?
   _____ A. Crista galli
   _____ B. Vomer
   _____ C. Orbital plate of frontal bone
   _____ D. Cribriform plate

4. Which number illustrates the inferior concha?
   _____ A. 10
   _____ B. 9
   _____ C. 7
   _____ D. 4

5. Which number illustrates the ethmoid sinus?
   _____ A. 9
   _____ B. 10
   _____ C. 8
   _____ D. 4

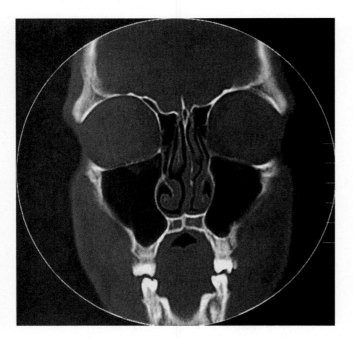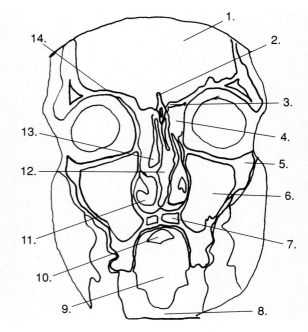

Figure 5-26

1. Which of the following is illustrated by 6?
   _____ A. Sphenoid sinus
   _____ B. Ethmoid sinus
   _____ C. Maxillary sinus
   _____ D. Frontal sinus

2. Which of the following is illustrated by 13?
   _____ A. Superior concha
   _____ B. Middle concha
   _____ C. Inferior concha
   _____ D. Nasal septum

3. Which of the following is illustrated by 5?
   _____ A. Ethmoid
   _____ B. Zygoma
   _____ C. Maxilla
   _____ D. Palatine

4. Which number illustrates the cribriform plate?
   _____ A. 2
   _____ B. 3
   _____ C. 14
   _____ D. 7

5. Which number illustrates the crista galli?
   _____ A. 2
   _____ B. 3
   _____ C. 4
   _____ D. 14

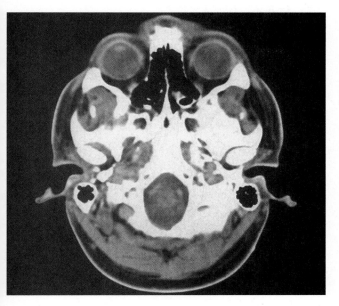
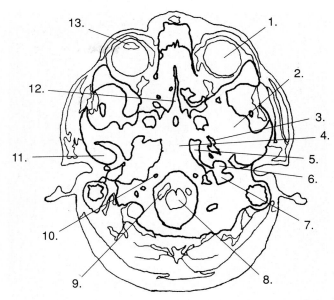

Figure 5-27

1. Which number illustrates the foramen ovale?
_____ A. 5
_____ B. 3
_____ C. 6
_____ D. 7

2. Which of the following is illustrated by 7?
_____ A. Internal jugular vein
_____ B. Foramen lacerum
_____ C. Foramen ovale
_____ D. Internal carotid artery

3. Which number illustrates the hypoglossal canal?
_____ A. 6
_____ B. 7
_____ C. 10
_____ D. 5

4. Which of the following illustrates the foramen lacerum?
_____ A. 7
_____ B. 6
_____ C. 10
_____ D. 5

5. Which of the following is illustrated by 6?
_____ A. Foramen lacerum
_____ B. Internal carotid artery
_____ C. Foramen ovale
_____ D. Internal jugular vein

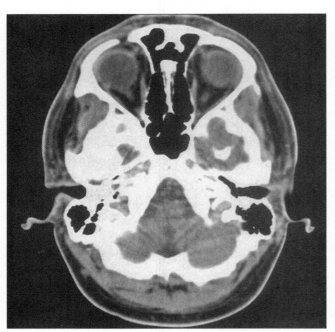
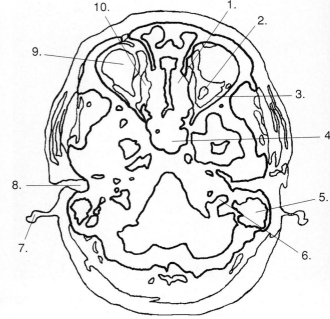

Figure 5-28

1. Which of the following is illustrated by 3?
   _____ A. Lateral rectus muscle
   _____ B. Medial rectus muscle
   _____ C. Optic nerve
   _____ D. Superior oblique muscle

2. Which number illustrates the ethmoid air cells?
   _____ A. 4
   _____ B. 1
   _____ C. 8
   _____ D. 5

3. Which number illustrates the medial rectus muscle?
   _____ A. 10
   _____ B. 3
   _____ C. 1
   _____ D. 2

4. Which of the following is illustrated by 5?
   _____ A. Temporal lobe
   _____ B. Sigmoid sinus
   _____ C. Internal carotid artery
   _____ D. Mastoid air cells

5. Which of the following is illustrated by 8?
   _____ A. Auricle
   _____ B. External acoustic meatus
   _____ C. Mandibular condyle
   _____ D. Hypoglossal canal

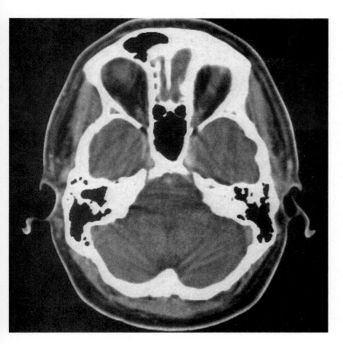
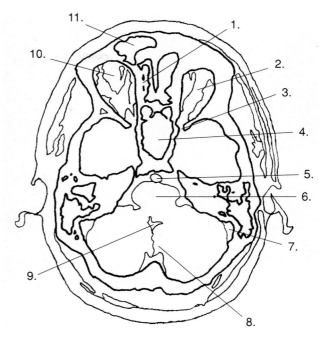

Figure 5-29

1. Which number illustrates the cribriform plate of the ethmoid bone?
   _____ A. 2
   _____ B. 11
   _____ C. 4
   _____ D. 1

2. Which of the following is illustrated by 6?
   _____ A. Pons
   _____ B. Medulla oblongata
   _____ C. Cerebellar vermis
   _____ D. Cerebral peduncles

3. Which number illustrates the basilar artery?
   _____ A. 6
   _____ B. 4
   _____ C. 5
   _____ D. 9

4. Which of the following is illustrated by 9?
   _____ A. Fourth ventricle
   _____ B. Basilar artery
   _____ C. Superior cistern
   _____ D. Inferior sagittal sinus

5. Which of the following is illustrated by 4?
   _____ A. Ethmoid air cells
   _____ B. Mastoid air cells
   _____ C. Sigmoid sinus
   _____ D. Sphenoid sinus

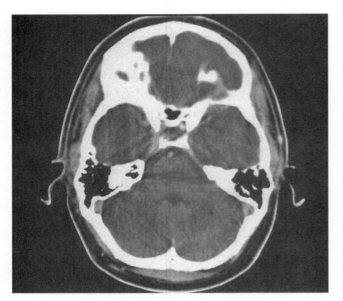

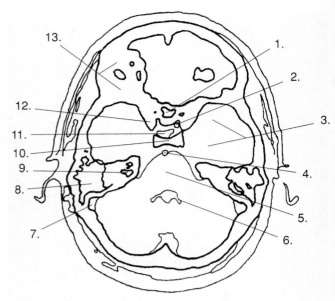

Figure 5-30

1. Which number illustrates the dorsum sellae?
    _____ A. 12
    _____ B. 10
    _____ C. 3
    _____ D. 11

2. Which of the following is illustrated by 1?
    _____ A. Optic chiasma
    _____ B. Internal carotid artery
    _____ C. Basilar artery
    _____ D. Sphenoid sinus

3. Which number illustrates the middle ear?
    _____ A. 4
    _____ B. 11
    _____ C. 9
    _____ D. 10

4. Which of the following is illustrated by 4?
    _____ A. Basilar artery
    _____ B. Interior carotid artery
    _____ C. Middle ear
    _____ D. Pituitary gland

5. Which of the following is illustrated by 11?
    _____ A. Pituitary gland
    _____ B. Dorsum sellae
    _____ C. Optic chiasma
    _____ D. Pineal gland

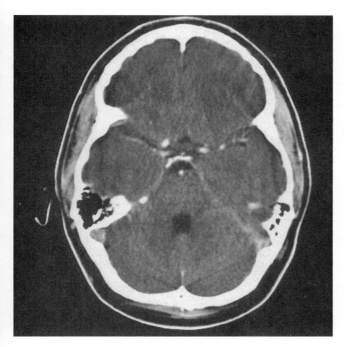
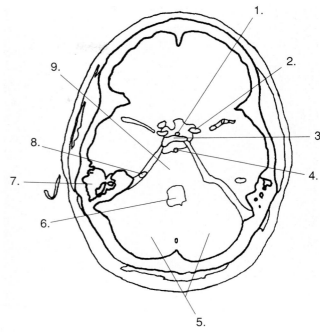

Figure 5-31

1. Which number illustrates the infundibulum of the pituitary?
   _____ A. 2
   _____ B. 4
   _____ C. 8
   _____ D. 1

2. Which of the following is illustrated by 3?
   _____ A. Basilar artery
   _____ B. Middle cerebral artery
   _____ C. Posterior cerebral artery
   _____ D. Dorsum sellae

3. Which number illustrates the mastoid air cells?
   _____ A. 7
   _____ B. 6
   _____ C. 3
   _____ D. 8

4. Which of the following is illustrated by 2?
   _____ A. Infundibulum of the pituitary
   _____ B. Middle cerebral artery
   _____ C. Anterior cerebral artery
   _____ D. Basilar artery

5. Which number illustrates the posterior cerebral artery?
   _____ A. 8
   _____ B. 6
   _____ C. 1
   _____ D. 4

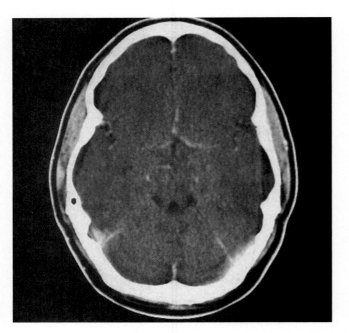

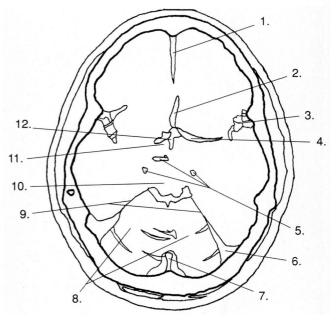

Figure 5-32

1. Which of the following is illustrated by 9?
   _____ A. Midbrain
   _____ B. Transverse sinus
   _____ C. Tentorium cerebelli
   _____ D. Cerebellum

2. Which number illustrates the falx cerebri?
   _____ A. 7
   _____ B. 2
   _____ C. 5
   _____ D. 1

3. Which of the following illustrates the hypothalamus?
   _____ A. 12
   _____ B. 11
   _____ C. 8
   _____ D. 10

4. Which number illustrates the Sylvian fissure?
   _____ A. 3
   _____ B. 1
   _____ C. 9
   _____ D. 12

5. Which of the following illustrates the falx cerebelli?
   _____ A. 1
   _____ B. 4
   _____ C. 7
   _____ D. 2

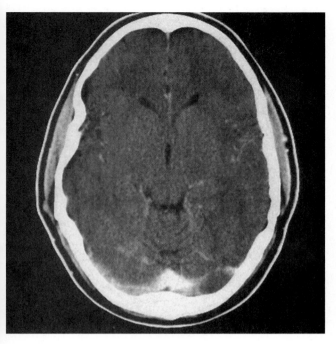 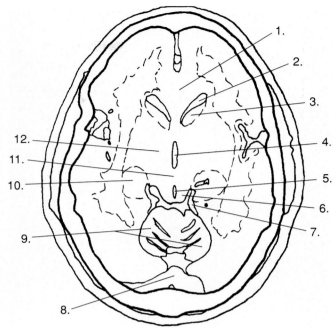

Figure 5-33

1. Which number illustrates the quadrigeminal plate?
   _____ A. 6
   _____ B. 2
   _____ C. 7
   _____ D. 3

2. Which number illustrates the cerebral peduncles?
   _____ A. 6
   _____ B. 11
   _____ C. 10
   _____ D. 12

3. Which of the following is illustrated by 4?
   _____ A. Fourth ventricle
   _____ B. Cerebral aqueduct
   _____ C. Third ventricle
   _____ D. Superior cistern

4. Which number illustrates the hippocampal formation?
   _____ A. 3
   _____ B. 6
   _____ C. 11
   _____ D. 10

5. Which number illustrates the posterior cerebral artery?
   _____ A. 7
   _____ B. 4
   _____ C. 8
   _____ D. 5

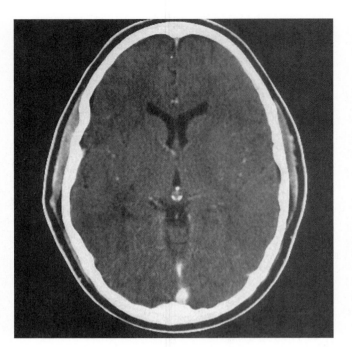
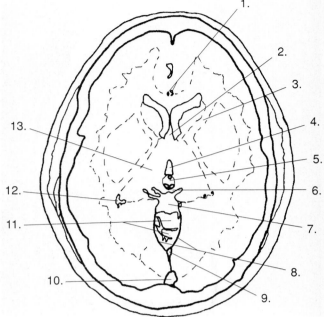

Figure 5-34

1. Which of the following is illustrated by 2?
   _____ A. Thalamus
   _____ B. Internal capsule
   _____ C. Fornix
   _____ D. Head of caudate

2. Which number illustrates the quadrigeminal plate?
   _____ A. 6
   _____ B. 8
   _____ C. 7
   _____ D. 11

3. Which number illustrates the inferior horn of the lateral ventricle?
   _____ A. 8
   _____ B. 5
   _____ C. 4
   _____ D. 12

4. Which of the following is illustrated by 9?
   _____ A. Confluence of sinuses
   _____ B. Straight sinus
   _____ C. Inferior sagittal sinus
   _____ D. Superior sagittal sinus

5. Which of the following is illustrated by 7?
   _____ A. Quadrigeminal plate
   _____ B. Superior cistern
   _____ C. Third ventricle
   _____ D. Straight sinus

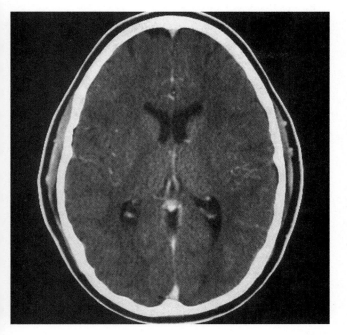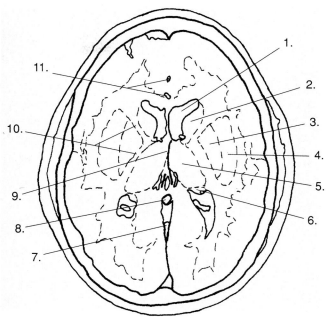

Figure 5-35

1. Which number illustrates the thalamus nucleus?
   _____ A. 2
   _____ B. 4
   _____ C. 3
   _____ D. 5

2. Which of the following is illustrated by 8?
   _____ A. Posterior cerebral artery
   _____ B. Vein of Galen
   _____ C. Third ventricle
   _____ D. Anterior cerebral artery

3. Which number illustrates the straight sinus?
   _____ A. 9
   _____ B. 6
   _____ C. 7
   _____ D. 1

4. Which of the following is illustrated by 4?
   _____ A. Head of caudate
   _____ B. Globus pallidus
   _____ C. Putamen
   _____ D. Tail of caudate

5. Which number illustrates the globus pallidus nucleus?
   _____ A. 2
   _____ B. 4
   _____ C. 3
   _____ D. 6

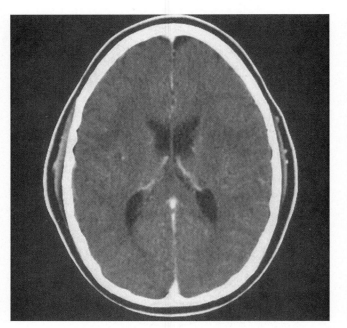 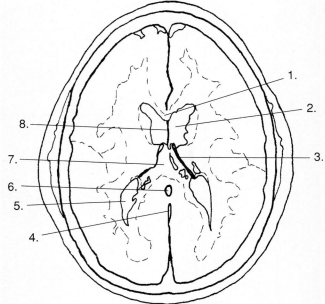

Figure 5-36

1. Which of the following is illustrated by 2?
   _____ A. Anterior horn of lateral ventricle
   _____ B. Body of lateral ventricle
   _____ C. Third ventricle
   _____ D. Superior cistern

2. Which number illustrates the septum pellucidum?
   _____ A. 1
   _____ B. 4
   _____ C. 3
   _____ D. 8

3. Which of the following is illustrated by 7?
   _____ A. Pons
   _____ B. Splenium of corpus callosum
   _____ C. Hypothalamus
   _____ D. Thalamus

4. Which number illustrates the posterior horn of the lateral ventricle?
   _____ A. 3
   _____ B. 6
   _____ C. 5
   _____ D. 2

5. Which of the following is illustrated by 3?
   _____ A. Posterior horn of the lateral ventricle
   _____ B. Choroid plexus
   _____ C. Splenium of corpus callosum
   _____ D. Septum pellucidum

CLINICAL APPLICATIONS

1. What bones form the bony nasal septum?

   _____

   _____

   _____

2. Which of the following nuclei appears to be protruding into the lateral ventricles?
   _____ A. Putamen
   _____ B. Caudate
   _____ C. Globus pallidus
   _____ D. Thalamus

3. Describe the location of the insula.

   _____

   _____

   _____

4. Which of the following describes the venous sinus between the inferior margin of the falx cerebri and tentorium cerebelli?
   _____ A. Superior sagittal sinus
   _____ B. Sigmoid sinus
   _____ C. Straight sinus
   _____ D. Inferior sagittal sinus

5. Describe the fornix.

   _____

   _____

   _____

6. Which of the following is most laterally situated within the brain?
   _____ A. Putamen
   _____ B. Caudate
   _____ C. Globus pallidus
   _____ D. Thalamus

7. The _____ transmits cerebrospinal fluid between the third and fourth ventricles.
   _____ A. Foramen of Magendie
   _____ B. Interventricular foramen
   _____ C. Foramen of Luschka
   _____ D. Cerebral aqueduct

8. The vertebral arteries enter the cranial cavity through the foramen _____.

9. Which of the following sinuses is located most posteriorly within the skull?
   _____ A. Sphenoid
   _____ B. Maxillary
   _____ C. Ethmoid
   _____ D. Frontal

10. Which of the following is found closest to the clivus?
   _____ A. Pons
   _____ B. Midbrain
   _____ C. Medulla oblongata
   _____ D. Hypothalamus

CLINICAL CORRELATIONS

■ Clinical Case 5-1

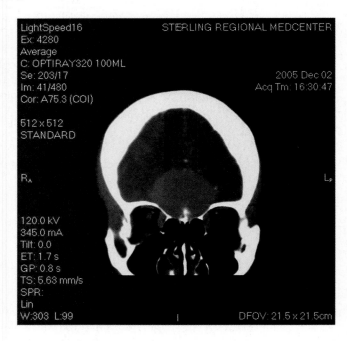

1. Which of the following describes the artery located superior to the cerebellum?
   _____ A. Posterior cerebral
   _____ B. Anterior cerebral
   _____ C. Middle cerebral
   _____ D. Basilar artery

2. In this patient, the location of the mass would best be described by which of the following:
   _____ A. Anterior cranial fossa
   _____ B. Middle cranial fossa
   _____ C. Posterior cranial fossa
   _____ D. Midbrain

3. Which of the following best describes the changes in adjacent tissues?
   _____ A. Inferior displacement of the pons
   _____ B. Superior displacement of the occipital lobe
   _____ C. Lateral displacement of the temporal lobe
   _____ D. Superior displacement of the frontal lobe

4. Which of the following describes the artery located anterior to the pons?
   _____ A. Posterior cerebral
   _____ B. Anterior cerebral
   _____ C. Middle cerebral
   _____ D. Basilar artery

5. Which of the following would best describe the procedure used to generate the images located above?
   _____ A. Computed tomography angiography (CTA)
   _____ B. Magnetic resonance angiography (MRA)
   _____ C. Ultrasound
   _____ D. Positron emission tomography/computed tomography (PET/CT)

■ Clinical Case 5-2

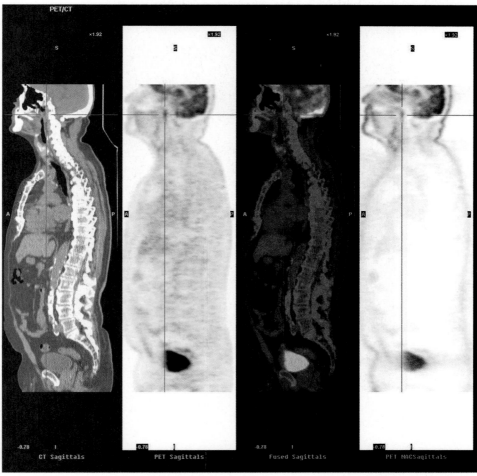

1. Which of the following best describes the location of the mass marked above?
   _____ A. Retropharyngeal
   _____ B. Oropharynx
   _____ C. Laryngopharynx
   _____ D. Retroperitoneal

2. The opening in the base of the skull that transmits the internal carotid artery is found in which of the following bones?
   _____ A. Sphenoid
   _____ B. Temporal
   _____ C. Frontal
   _____ D. Occipital

3. The opening in the base of the skull that transmits the internal jugular vein is found in which of the following bones?
   _____ A. Sphenoid
   _____ B. Temporal
   _____ C. Frontal
   _____ D. Occipital

4. Which of the following is the foramen that contains the vertebral arteries?
   _____ A. Ovale
   _____ B. Lacerum
   _____ C. Magnum
   _____ D. Superior orbital fissure

5. Which of the cranial nerves exits the skull to carry sensory and motor fibers below the diaphragm?
   _____ A. Hypoglossal
   _____ B. Trochlear
   _____ C. Vagus
   _____ D. Trigeminal

■ Clinical Case 5-3

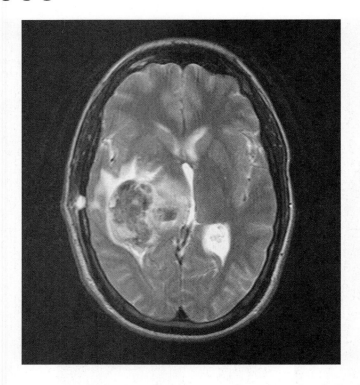

1. Describe the location of the glioblastoma multiforme in this axial, contrast-enhanced magnetic resonance (MR) image of the brain.

   _____

   _____

   _____

2. Describe the changes in adjacent tissues.

   _____

   _____

   _____

3. Describe the consistency, shape, and border.

   _____

   _____

   _____

■ Clinical Case 5-4

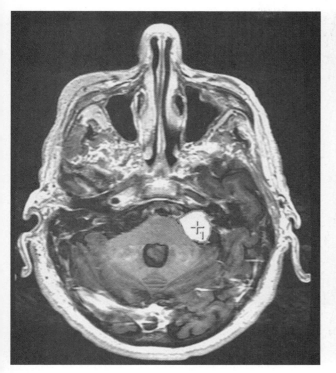 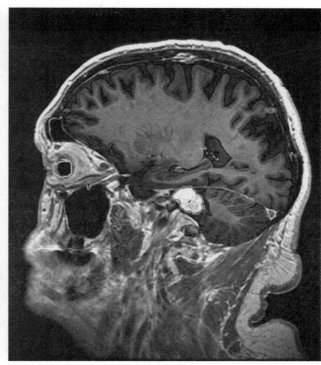

1. Describe the location of the acoustic neuroma in the axial (left) and sagittal (right) T1 weighted MR images in this 80-year-old male patient.

   _____

   _____

   _____

2. Describe the changes in adjacent tissues.

   _____

   _____

   _____

3. Describe the consistency, shape, and border.

   _____

   _____

   _____

■ Clinical Case 5-5

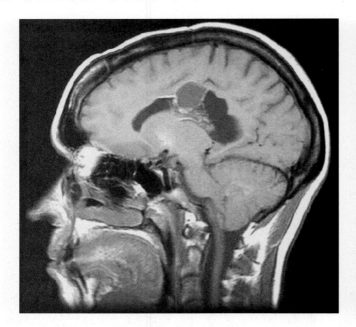 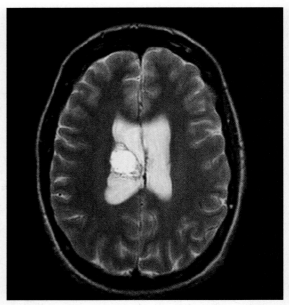

1. Describe the location of the neurocytoma shown in the sagittal T1 (left) and axial T2 (right) weighted MR images of the head.

   _____

   _____

   _____

2. Describe the changes in adjacent tissues.

   _____

   _____

   _____

3. Describe the consistency, shape, and border.

   _____

   _____

   _____

■ Clinical Case 5-6

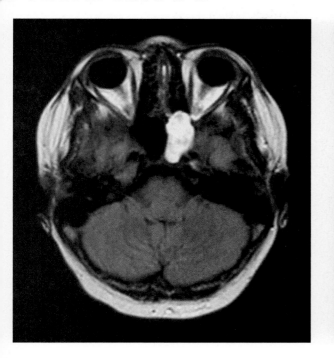 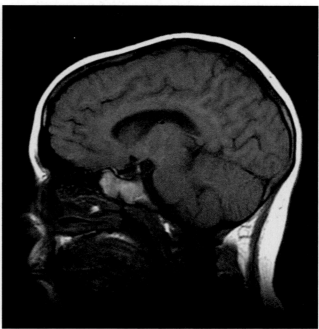

1. Describe the location of the mucocele shown in the T1 weighted axial and sagittal MR images.

   _____

   _____

   _____

2. Describe the changes in adjacent tissues.

   _____

   _____

   _____

3. Describe the consistency, shape, and border.

   _____

   _____

   _____

■ Clinical Case 5-7

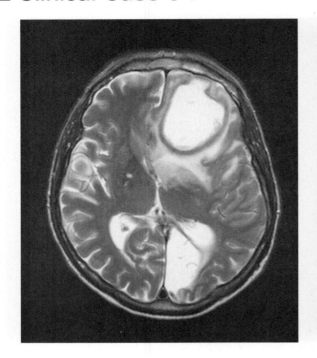 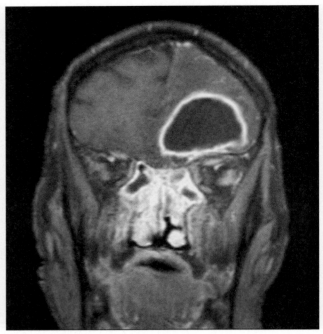

1. Describe the location of the brain abscess shown on the axial T2 (left) and coronal T1 (right) weighted post contrast MR images.

   _____

   _____

   _____

2. Describe the changes in adjacent tissues.

   _____

   _____

   _____

3. Describe the consistency, shape, and border.

   _____

   _____

   _____

■ Clinical Case 5-8

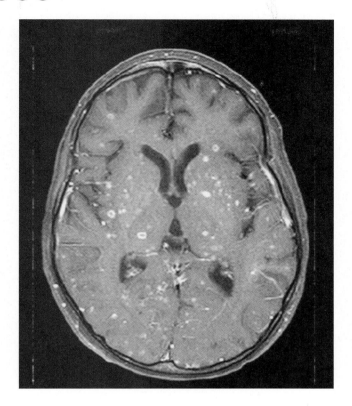

1. Describe the location of the infection in this axial MR brain image of a 14-year-old female patient.

   _____

   _____

   _____

2. Describe the changes in adjacent tissues.

   _____

   _____

   _____

3. Describe the consistency, shape, and border.

   _____

   _____

   _____

Chapter 6 Neck

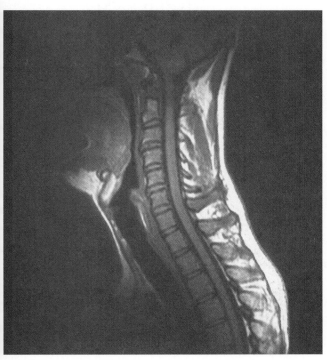

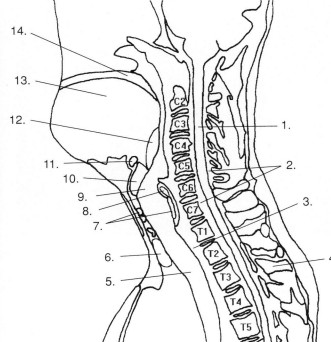

Figure 6-1

1. Which of the following is illustrated by 14?
   _____ A. Nasopharynx
   _____ B. Genioglossus muscle
   _____ C. Soft palate
   _____ D. Maxilla

2. Which of the following is illustrated by 7?
   _____ A. Thyroid cartilage
   _____ B. Cricoid cartilage
   _____ C. Arytenoid cartilage
   _____ D. Hyoid bone

3. Which number illustrates the genioglossus muscle?
   _____ A. 13
   _____ B. 14
   _____ C. 12
   _____ D. 10

4. Which of the following is illustrated by 8?
   _____ A. Arytenoid cartilage
   _____ B. Cricoid cartilage
   _____ C. Thyroid cartilage
   _____ D. Hyoid bone

5. Which number illustrates the isthmus of the thyroid gland?
   _____ A. 12
   _____ B. 7
   _____ C. 10
   _____ D. 6

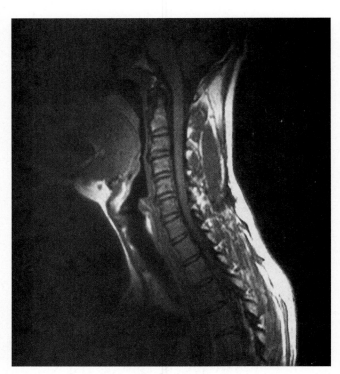

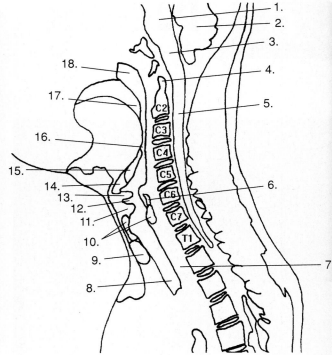

Figure 6-2

1. Which number illustrates the vestibular fold?
   _____ A. 13
   _____ B. 6
   _____ C. 11
   _____ D. 18

2. Which of the following is illustrated by 15?
   _____ A. Oropharynx
   _____ B. Epiglottis
   _____ C. Cricoid cartilage
   _____ D. Arytenoid cartilage

3. Which of the following is illustrated by 12?
   _____ A. Vestibular fold
   _____ B. Uvula
   _____ C. Laryngeal pharynx
   _____ D. Glottic space

4. Which number illustrates the thyroid cartilage?
   _____ A. 14
   _____ B. 15
   _____ C. 6
   _____ D. 10

5. Which number illustrates the vocal fold?
   _____ A. 12
   _____ B. 13
   _____ C. 11
   _____ D. 15

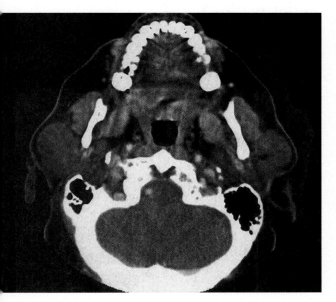
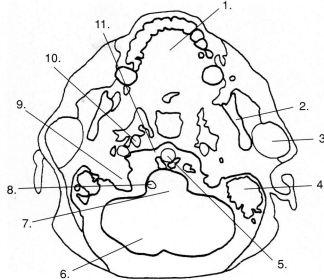

Figure 6-3

1. Which of the following is illustrated by 8?
   _____ A. Basilar artery
   _____ B. Posterior cerebral artery
   _____ C. Right vertebral artery
   _____ D. Right internal carotid artery

2. Which number illustrates the sigmoid sinus?
   _____ A. 9
   _____ B. 10
   _____ C. 4
   _____ D. 5

3. Which of the following is illustrated by 3?
   _____ A. Submandibular gland
   _____ B. Mastoid air cells
   _____ C. Ramus of the mandible
   _____ D. Parotid gland

4. Which number illustrates the internal carotid artery?
   _____ A. 5
   _____ B. 9
   _____ C. 10
   _____ D. 8

5. Which of the following is illustrated by 11?
   _____ A. Occipital bone
   _____ B. Dens
   _____ C. Styloid process
   _____ D. Anterior arch of the atlas

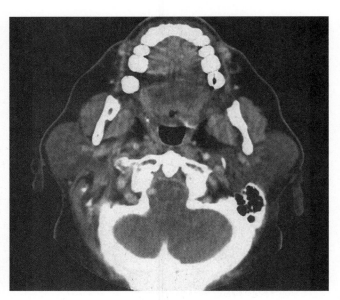 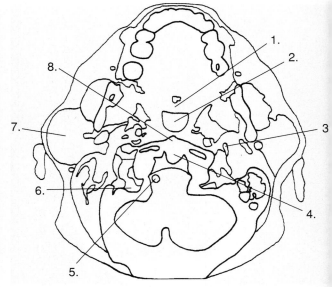

Figure 6-4

1. Which of the following is illustrated by 3?
   _____ A. Internal carotid artery
   _____ B. Styloid process
   _____ C. Internal jugular vein
   _____ D. Dens

2. Which number illustrates the internal jugular vein?
   _____ A. 6
   _____ B. 5
   _____ C. 2
   _____ D. 3

3. Which of the following is illustrated by 7?
   _____ A. Retromandibular vein
   _____ B. Submandibular gland
   _____ C. Parotid gland
   _____ D. Sublingual gland

4. Which of the following is illustrated by 2?
   _____ A. Vallecula
   _____ B. Laryngeal pharynx
   _____ C. Uvula
   _____ D. Oropharynx

5. Which of the following is illustrated by 5?
   _____ A. Basilar artery
   _____ B. Internal jugular vein
   _____ C. Vertebral artery
   _____ D. Internal carotid artery

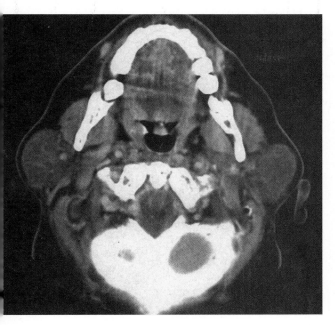

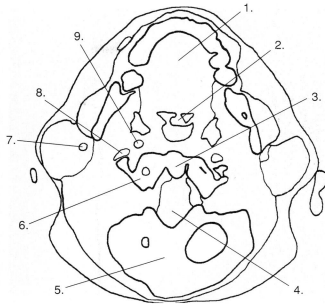

Figure 6-5

1. Which number illustrates the uvula?
   _____ A. 6
   _____ B. 2
   _____ C. 4
   _____ D. 3

2. Which of the following is illustrated by 7?
   _____ A. Parotid gland
   _____ B. Right retromandibular vein
   _____ C. External jugular vein
   _____ D. Internal jugular vein

3. Which of the following is illustrated by 1?
   _____ A. Soft palate
   _____ B. Geniohyoid
   _____ C. Sternocleidomastoid
   _____ D. Genioglossus muscle

4. Which of the following is illustrated by 6?
   _____ A. Atlas
   _____ B. Dens
   _____ C. Axis
   _____ D. Occipital bone

5. Which of the following is illustrated by 4?
   _____ A. Spinal cord
   _____ B. Pons
   _____ C. Cerebral peduncles
   _____ D. Oropharynx

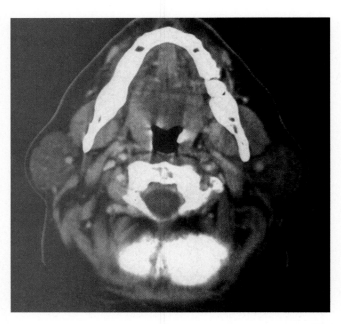

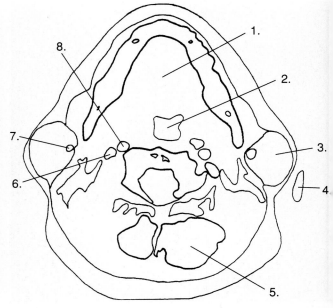

Figure 6-6

1. Which number illustrates the oropharynx?
   _____ A. 8
   _____ B. 4
   _____ C. 2
   _____ D. 3

2. Which of the following is illustrated by 3?
   _____ A. Submandibular gland
   _____ B. Sublingual gland
   _____ C. Uvula
   _____ D. Parotid gland

3. Which number illustrates the internal jugular vein?
   _____ A. 6
   _____ B. 2
   _____ C. 8
   _____ D. 7

4. Which of the following is illustrated by 8?
   _____ A. Internal jugular vein
   _____ B. Retromandibular vein
   _____ C. Vertebral artery
   _____ D. Internal carotid artery

5. Which of the following is illustrated by 5?
   _____ A. Dens
   _____ B. Atlas
   _____ C. Occipital bone
   _____ D. Axis

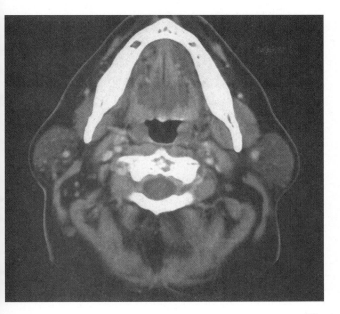
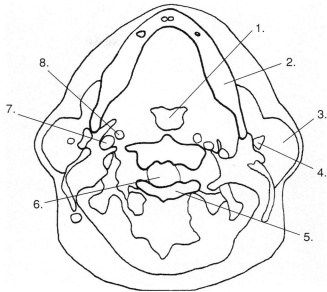

Figure 6-7

1. Which of the following is illustrated by 2?
  _____ A. Maxilla
  _____ B. Ramus of mandible
  _____ C. Body of mandible
  _____ D. Coronoid notch

2. Which number illustrates the lamina?
  _____ A. 5
  _____ B. 6
  _____ C. 2
  _____ D. 4

3. Which of the following is illustrated by 4?
  _____ A. Right retromandibular vein
  _____ B. Left retromandibular vein
  _____ C. Right external jugular vein
  _____ D. Left external jugular vein

4. Which number illustrates the parotid gland?
  _____ A. 1
  _____ B. 6
  _____ C. 5
  _____ D. 3

5. Which number illustrates the internal carotid artery?
  _____ A. 8
  _____ B. 4
  _____ C. 7
  _____ D. 6

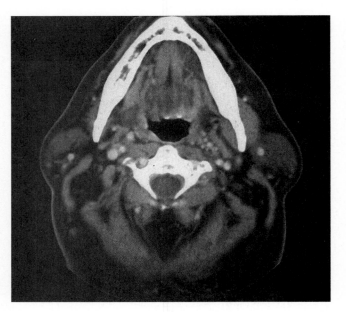
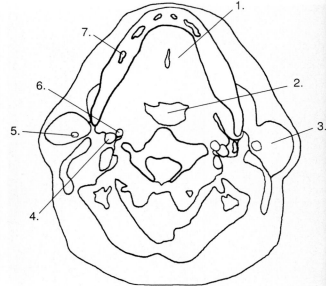

Figure 6-8

1. Which of the following is illustrated by 4?
   _____ A. Right internal carotid artery
   _____ B. Left internal carotid artery
   _____ C. Right internal jugular vein
   _____ D. Left internal jugular vein

2. Which of the following is illustrated by 1?
   _____ A. Soft palate
   _____ B. Geniohyoid muscle
   _____ C. Sternocleidomastoid muscle
   _____ D. Genioglossus muscle

3. Which of the following is illustrated by 7?
   _____ A. Body of mandible
   _____ B. Ramus of mandible
   _____ C. Maxilla
   _____ D. Coronoid notch

4. Which of the following is illustrated by 6?
   _____ A. Right internal jugular vein
   _____ B. Left internal jugular vein
   _____ C. Right internal carotid artery
   _____ D. Left retromandibular vein

5. Which of the following is illustrated by 5?
   _____ A. Right internal carotid artery
   _____ B. Left internal carotid artery
   _____ C. Left retromandibular vein
   _____ D. Right retromandibular vein

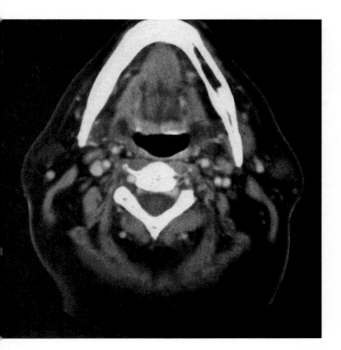

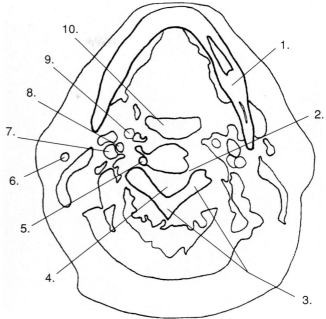

Figure 6-9

1. Which of the following illustrates the intervertebral foramen?
   _____ A. 4
   _____ B. 3
   _____ C. 2
   _____ D. 10

2. Which number illustrates the internal jugular vein?
   _____ A. 7
   _____ B. 8
   _____ C. 6
   _____ D. 5

3. Which of the following is illustrated by 5?
   _____ A. Internal carotid artery
   _____ B. Internal jugular vein
   _____ C. Retromandibular vein
   _____ D. Vertebral artery

4. Which of the following is illustrated by 4?
   _____ A. Lamina
   _____ B. Spinal cord
   _____ C. Intervertebral foramen
   _____ D. Oropharynx

5. Which of the following is illustrated by 9?
   _____ A. Internal carotid artery
   _____ B. Internal jugular vein
   _____ C. External carotid artery
   _____ D. Vertebral artery

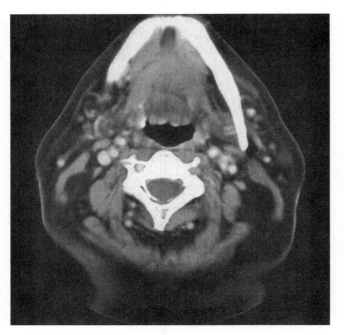
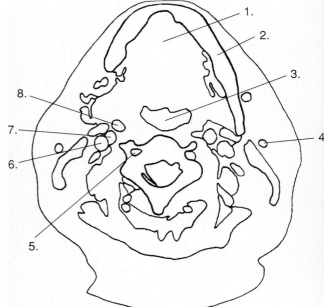

Figure 6-10

1. Which of the following is illustrated by 7?
   _____ A. Right internal carotid artery
   _____ B. Left internal carotid artery
   _____ C. Right external carotid artery
   _____ D. Left external carotid artery

2. Which number illustrates the body of the mandible?
   _____ A. 3
   _____ B. 1
   _____ C. 2
   _____ D. 8

3. Which of the following is illustrated by 3?
   _____ A. Larynx
   _____ B. Laryngeal pharynx
   _____ C. Nasopharynx
   _____ D. Oropharynx

4. Which of the following is illustrated by 6?
   _____ A. Internal carotid artery
   _____ B. External carotid artery
   _____ C. Internal jugular vein
   _____ D. External jugular vein

5. Which of the following is illustrated by 4?
   _____ A. Retromandibular vein
   _____ B. Retromandibular artery
   _____ C. External jugular vein
   _____ D. External carotid artery

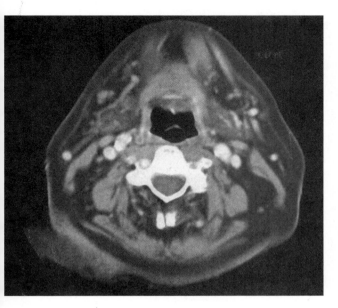 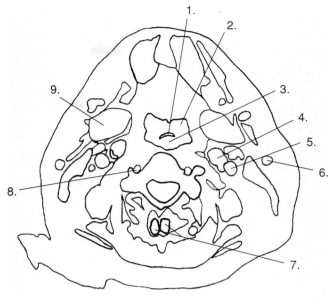

Figure 6-11

1. Which of the following is illustrated by 4?
    _____ A. Internal carotid artery
    _____ B. Common carotid artery
    _____ C. External jugular vein
    _____ D. Internal jugular vein

2. Which number illustrates the epiglottis?
    _____ A. 7
    _____ B. 9
    _____ C. 1
    _____ D. 8

3. Which number illustrates the internal jugular vein?
    _____ A. 5
    _____ B. 4
    _____ C. 6
    _____ D. 8

4. Which of the following is illustrated by 3?
    _____ A. Oropharynx
    _____ B. Laryngeal pharynx
    _____ C. Piriform sinus
    _____ D. Vallecula

5. Which of the following is illustrated by 2?
    _____ A. Vallecula
    _____ B. Glottic space
    _____ C. Laryngeal pharynx
    _____ D. Piriform sinus

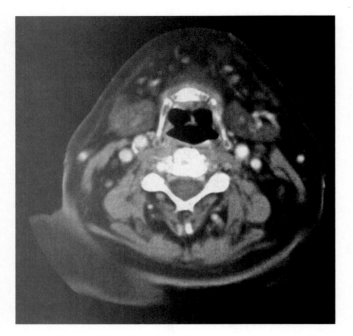

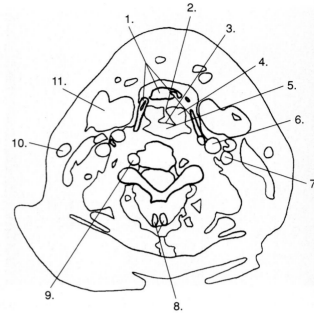

Figure 6-12

1. Which of the following is illustrated by 4?
   _____ A. Glottic space
   _____ B. Laryngeal pharynx
   _____ C. Piriform sinus
   _____ D. Vallecula

2. Which number illustrates the laryngeal pharynx?
   _____ A. 6
   _____ B. 4
   _____ C. 5
   _____ D. 3

3. Which number illustrates the median glossoepiglottic fold?
   _____ A. 3
   _____ B. 2
   _____ C. 11
   _____ D. 4

4. Which of the following is illustrated by 1?
   _____ A. Hyoid bone
   _____ B. Cricoid cartilage
   _____ C. Body of mandible
   _____ D. Thyroid cartilage

5. Which of the following is illustrated by 7?
   _____ A. Common carotid artery
   _____ B. Internal carotid artery
   _____ C. Internal jugular vein
   _____ D. External jugular vein

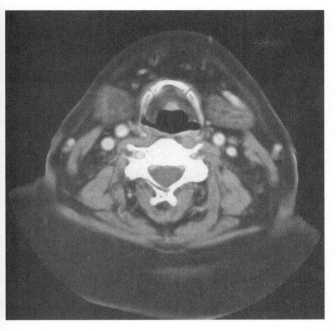
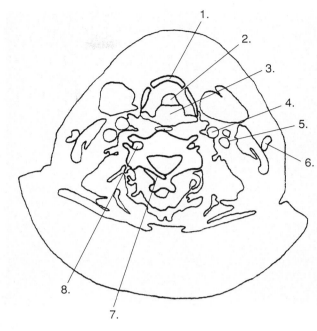

Figure 6-13

1. Which of the following is illustrated by 6?
   _____ A. External jugular vein
   _____ B. Internal jugular vein
   _____ C. Retromandibular vein
   _____ D. External carotid artery

2. Which number illustrates the laryngeal vestibule?
   _____ A. 2
   _____ B. 3
   _____ C. 1
   _____ D. 8

3. Which of the following is illustrated by 2?
   _____ A. Arytenoid cartilage
   _____ B. Uvula
   _____ C. Epiglottis
   _____ D. Laryngeal vestibule

4. Which of the following is illustrated by 4?
   _____ A. Internal jugular vein
   _____ B. Internal carotid artery
   _____ C. Common carotid artery
   _____ D. External jugular vein

5. Which of the following is illustrated by 1?
   _____ A. Cricoid cartilage
   _____ B. Arytenoid cartilage
   _____ C. Thyroid cartilage
   _____ D. Hyoid bone

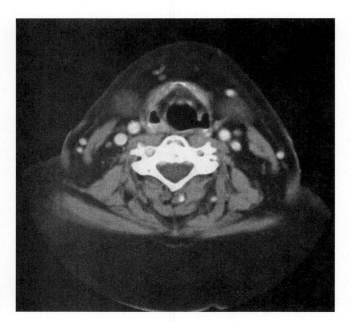

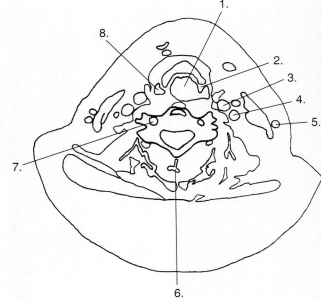

Figure 6-14

1. Which number illustrates the vertebral artery?
   _____ A. 3
   _____ B. 4
   _____ C. 7
   _____ D. 5

2. Which of the following is illustrated by 1?
   _____ A. Piriform sinus
   _____ B. Laryngeal vestibule
   _____ C. Vallecula
   _____ D. Laryngeal pharynx

3. Which of the following is illustrated by 8?
   _____ A. Vallecula
   _____ B. Laryngeal pharynx
   _____ C. Piriform sinus
   _____ D. Laryngeal vestibule

4. Which of the following is illustrated by 2?
   _____ A. Aryepiglottic fold
   _____ B. Vestibular fold
   _____ C. Vallecula
   _____ D. Vocal fold

5. Which number illustrates the common carotid artery?
   _____ A. 7
   _____ B. 5
   _____ C. 4
   _____ D. 3

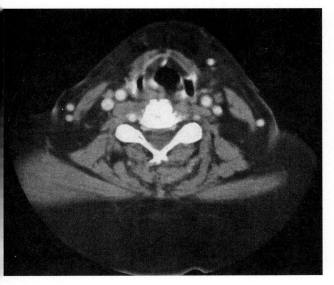 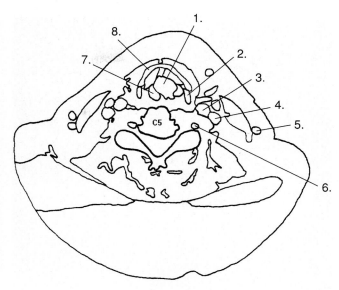

Figure 6-15

1. Which of the following is illustrated by 6?
   _____ A. Vertebral artery
   _____ B. External jugular vein
   _____ C. Internal jugular vein
   _____ D. Common carotid artery

2. Which of the following is illustrated by 8?
   _____ A. Cricoid cartilage
   _____ B. Thyroid cartilage
   _____ C. Hyoid bone
   _____ D. Arytenoid cartilage

3. Which number illustrates the laryngeal vestibule?
   _____ A. 8
   _____ B. 7
   _____ C. 1
   _____ D. 2

4. Which number illustrates the piriform sinus?
   _____ A. 2
   _____ B. 7
   _____ C. 8
   _____ D. 1

5. Which of the following is illustrated by 7?
   _____ A. Vallecula
   _____ B. Thyroid cartilage
   _____ C. Laryngeal vestibule
   _____ D. Arytenoid cartilage

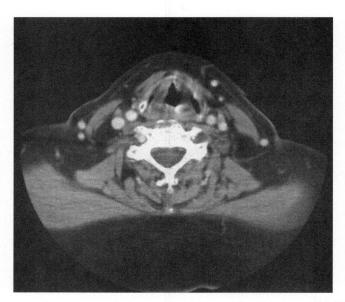
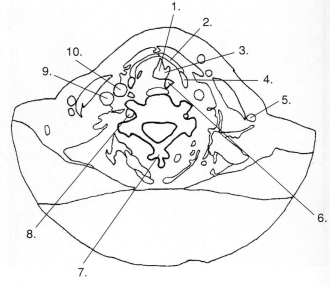

Figure 6-16

1. Which of the following is illustrated by 2?
    _____ A. Hyoid bone
    _____ B. Arytenoid cartilage
    _____ C. Cricoid cartilage
    _____ D. Thyroid cartilage

2. Which of the following is illustrated by 4?
    _____ A. Piriform sinus
    _____ B. Glottic space
    _____ C. Vallecula
    _____ D. Oropharynx

3. Which number illustrates the arytenoid cartilage?
    _____ A. 6
    _____ B. 2
    _____ C. 3
    _____ D. 4

4. Which of the following is illustrated by 3?
    _____ A. Oropharynx
    _____ B. Glottic space
    _____ C. Arytenoid cartilage
    _____ D. Laryngeal vestibule

5. Which number illustrates the common carotid artery?
    _____ A. 5
    _____ B. 8
    _____ C. 9
    _____ D. 10

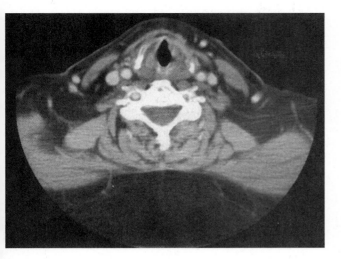
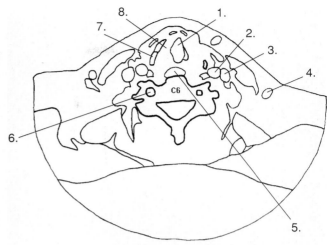

Figure 6-17

1. Which number illustrates the vocal cord?

_____ A. 5
_____ B. 7
_____ C. 8
_____ D. 1

2. Which of the following is illustrated by 5?

_____ A. Esophagus
_____ B. Thyroid cartilage
_____ C. Retropharynx
_____ D. Vocal cord

3. Which number illustrates the common carotid artery?

_____ A. 6
_____ B. 2
_____ C. 3
_____ D. 4

4. Which of the following is illustrated by 1?

_____ A. Vocal cord
_____ B. Glottic space
_____ C. Vallecula
_____ D. Infraglottic space

5. Which of the following is illustrated by 7?

_____ A. Hyoid bone
_____ B. Thyroid cartilage
_____ C. Cricoid cartilage
_____ D. Vocal cord

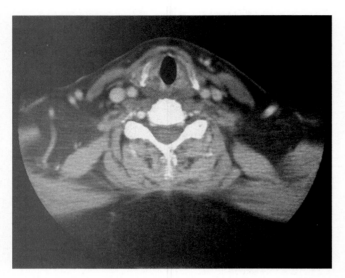 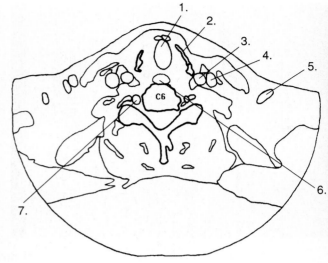

Figure 6-18

1. Which number illustrates the common carotid artery?
   _____ A. 3
   _____ B. 7
   _____ C. 4
   _____ D. 5

2. Which of the following is illustrated by 2?
   _____ A. Trachea
   _____ B. Arytenoid cartilage
   _____ C. Cricoid cartilage
   _____ D. Thyroid cartilage

3. Which of the following is illustrated by 6?
   _____ A. Thyroid cartilage
   _____ B. Trachea
   _____ C. Esophagus
   _____ D. Laryngeal vestibule

4. Which number illustrates the internal jugular vein?
   _____ A. 5
   _____ B. 7
   _____ C. 4
   _____ D. 3

5. Which of the following is illustrated by 1?
   _____ A. Trachea
   _____ B. Esophagus
   _____ C. Laryngeal vestibule
   _____ D. Laryngeal pharynx

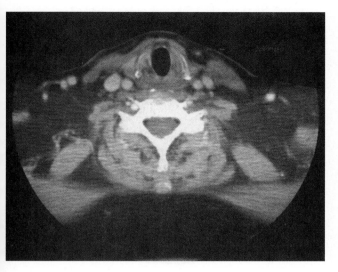
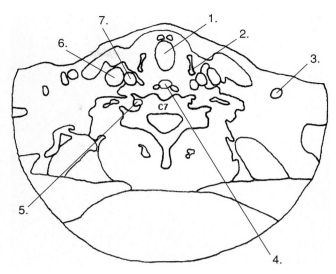

Figure 6-19

1. Which number illustrates the internal jugular vein?
    _____ A. 7
    _____ B. 5
    _____ C. 6
    _____ D. 3

2. Which of the following is illustrated by 6?
    _____ A. External jugular vein
    _____ B. Internal jugular vein
    _____ C. Retromandibular vein
    _____ D. Subclavian vein

3. Which of the following is illustrated by 2?
    _____ A. Thyroid cartilage
    _____ B. Cricoid cartilage
    _____ C. Arytenoid cartilage
    _____ D. Hyoid bone

4. Which of the following is illustrated by 4?
    _____ A. Trachea
    _____ B. Esophagus
    _____ C. Vallecula
    _____ D. Laryngeal pharynx

5. Which of the following is illustrated by 1?
    _____ A. Vallecula
    _____ B. Esophagus
    _____ C. Laryngeal pharynx
    _____ D. Trachea

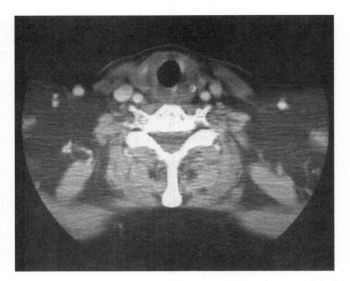

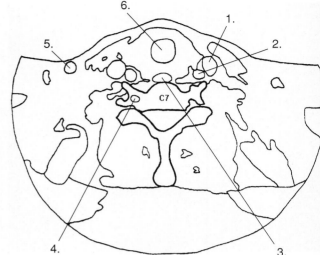

Figure 6-20

1. Which number illustrates the common carotid artery?
   _____ A. 1
   _____ B. 3
   _____ C. 4
   _____ D. 2

2. Which of the following is illustrated by 1?
   _____ A. External jugular vein
   _____ B. Internal jugular vein
   _____ C. Vertebral vein
   _____ D. Common carotid artery

3. Which number illustrates the external jugular vein?
   _____ A. 1
   _____ B. 4
   _____ C. 2
   _____ D. 5

4. Which of the following is illustrated by 6?
   _____ A. Infraglottic space
   _____ B. Glottic space
   _____ C. Trachea
   _____ D. Laryngeal vestibule

5. Which of the following is illustrated by 3?
   _____ A. Trachea
   _____ B. Laryngeal vestibule
   _____ C. Laryngeal pharynx
   _____ D. Esophagus

CLINICAL APPLICATIONS

1. C2 is also called the_____.

2. Which of the following vertebrae is described as not having a vertebral body?
   _____ A. Thoracic
   _____ B. Axis
   _____ C. C3 through C6
   _____ D. Atlas

3. Which of the following is described as a ring-shaped cartilage forming part of the larynx?
   _____ A. Arytenoid
   _____ B. Thyroid
   _____ C. Cricoid
   _____ D. Epiglottis

4. The vestibular folds are located superior to the vocal folds.
   True or false

5. The left vertebral artery originates from which of the following?
   _____ A. Aortic arch
   _____ B. Axillary artery
   _____ C. Subclavian artery
   _____ D. Common carotid artery

6. Describe the glottic space.

   _____

   _____

   _____

7. The aryepiglottic folds are also known as the false vocal cords.
   True or false

8. Which of the following vessels is located most anteriorly in the upper neck?
   _____ A. External carotid artery
   _____ B. Internal carotid artery
   _____ C. Internal jugular vein
   _____ D. Vertebral artery

9. The U-shaped _____ gland is located just below the larynx and has two large lobes on either side of the upper trachea.

10. The external jugular veins drain into the

    _____ veins on either side of the neck.

CLINICAL CORRELATIONS

■ Clinical Case 6-1

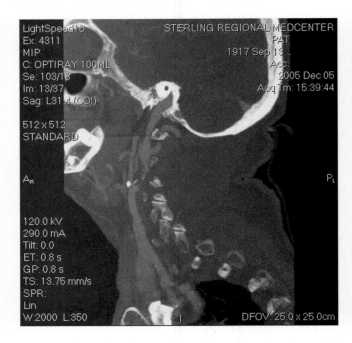
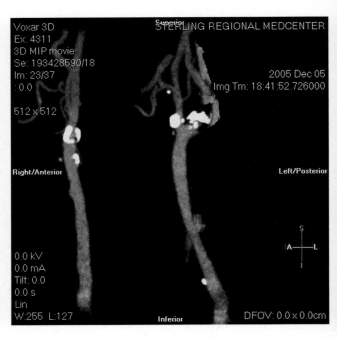

1. In the image above, which of the following best describes the location of the largest blockage?
   - _____ A. Origin of external carotid artery
   - _____ B. Origin of internal carotid artery
   - _____ C. Origin of right common iliac artery
   - _____ D. Origin of left common iliac artery

2. In this patient, the plaque causing greater arterial stenosis is found on which side?
   - _____ A. Right
   - _____ B. Left

3. In the sagittal image, which of the following vessels is shown entering the base of the skull?
   - _____ A. External carotid artery
   - _____ B. Internal carotid artery
   - _____ C. Right common iliac artery
   - _____ D. Left common iliac artery

4. Is the arterial blood flow within the vertebral artery demonstrated in any of the images above?
   - _____ A. No
   - _____ B. Yes

5. Is the arterial blood flow within the external carotid artery demonstrated in any of the images above?
   - _____ A. No
   - _____ B. Yes

■ Clinical Case 6-2

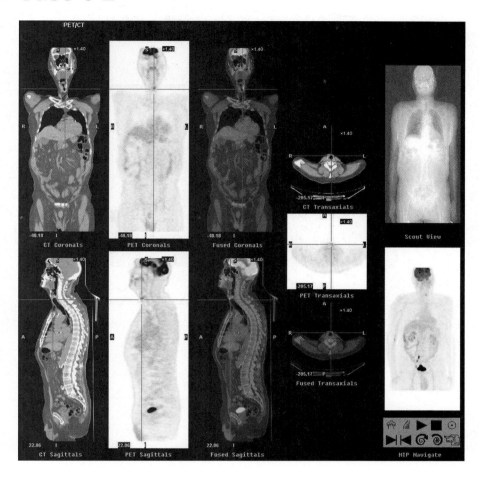

1. Which of the following best describes the location of the mass marked above?

_____ A. Retropharynx
_____ B. Oropharynx
_____ C. Laryngopharynx
_____ D. Larynx

2. In this patient, is the mass located on the right or left side?

_____ A. Right
_____ B. Left

3. Which of the following best describes the position of the mass as compared to the cricoid cartilage?

_____ A. Superior
_____ B. Inferior
_____ C. Lateral
_____ D. Medial

4. The vocal cords extend between which of the following cartilage structures?

_____ A. Thyroid to cricoid
_____ B. Cricoid to epiglottis
_____ C. Thyroid to arytenoid
_____ D. Arytenoid to cricoid

5. Which of the following best describes the position of the mass as compared to the epiglottis?

_____ A. Superior
_____ B. Inferior
_____ C. Lateral
_____ D. Medial

■ Clinical Case 6-3

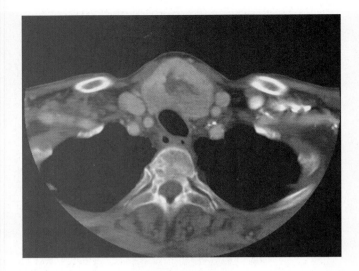

1. Describe the location of the thyroid adenoma in this axial computed tomography (CT) image.

   _____

   _____

   _____

2. Describe the changes in adjacent tissues.

   _____

   _____

   _____

3. Describe the consistency, shape, and border.

   _____

   _____

   _____

■ Clinical Case 6-4

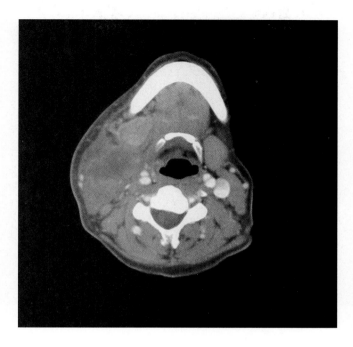

1. Describe the location of the mass in this axial CT section through the level of the hyoid bone.

   _____

   _____

   _____

2. Describe the changes in adjacent tissues.

   _____

   _____

   _____

3. Describe the consistency, shape, and border.

   _____

   _____

   _____

■ Clinical Case 6-5

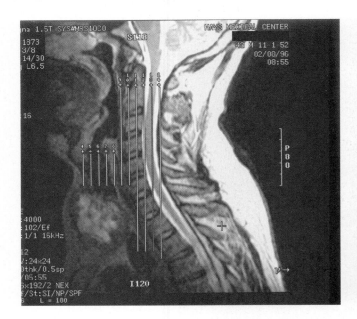 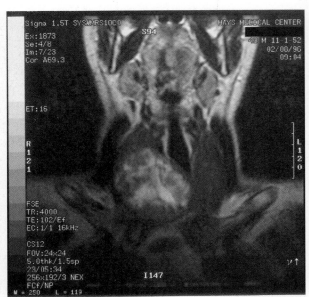

1. Describe the location of the carcinoma shown in the coronal (left) and sagittal (right) T2 weighted magnetic resonance (MR) images of this 43-year-old man.

    _____

    _____

    _____

2. Describe the changes in adjacent tissues.

    _____

    _____

    _____

3. Describe the consistency, shape, and border.

    _____

    _____

    _____

■ Clinical Case 6-6

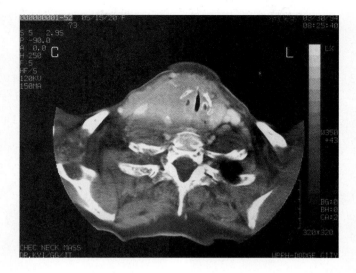

1. Describe the location of the lymphoma shown in this axial CT image of a 73-year-old female.

   _____

   _____

   _____

2. Describe the changes in adjacent tissues.

   _____

   _____

   _____

3. Describe the consistency, shape, and border.

   _____

   _____

   _____

■ Clinical Case 6-7

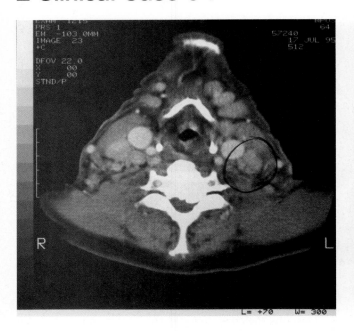 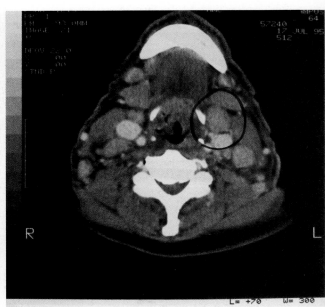

1. Describe the location of the adenopathy (enlarged lymph nodes circled) shown in the axial CT images following the administration of contrast to this 64-year-old patient previously diagnosed with Hodgkin disease.

   _____

   _____

   _____

2. Describe the changes in adjacent tissues.

   _____

   _____

   _____

3. Describe the consistency, shape, and border.

   _____

   _____

   _____

■ Clinical Case 6-8

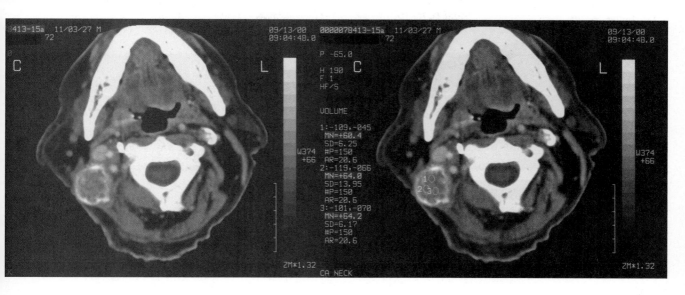

1. Describe the location of the parotid carcinoma in these contrast-enhanced axial CT sections through the neck at the level of the lower mandible in this 72-year-old male patient.

_____

_____

_____

2. Describe the changes in adjacent tissues.

_____

_____

_____

3. Describe the consistency, shape, and border.

_____

_____

_____

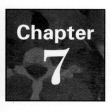
Spine

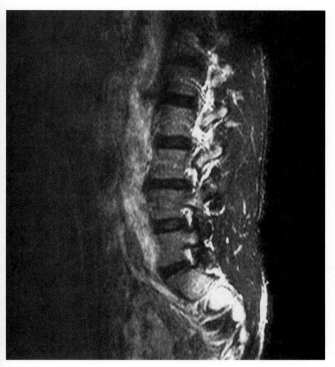

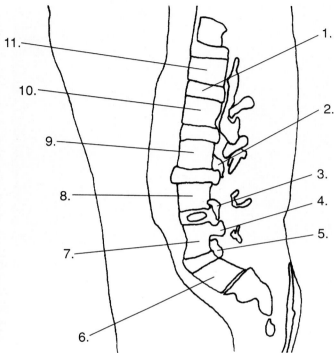

Figure 7-1

1. What number illustrates the pedicle?
   _____ A. 4
   _____ B. 2
   _____ C. 3
   _____ D. 5

2. Which of the following is illustrated by 8?
   _____ A. Vertebral body of L5
   _____ B. Intervertebral disk
   _____ C. Vertebral body of L4
   _____ D. L5 nerve roots

3. What number illustrates the vertebral body of S1?
   _____ A. 7
   _____ B. 8
   _____ C. 9
   _____ D. 6

4. Which of the following is illustrated by 1?
   _____ A. L3 nerve roots
   _____ B. Intervertebral disk
   _____ C. Vertebral body of L1
   _____ D. Pedicle of L5

5. What number illustrates the L5 nerve roots?
   _____ A. 6
   _____ B. 4
   _____ C. 5
   _____ D. 3

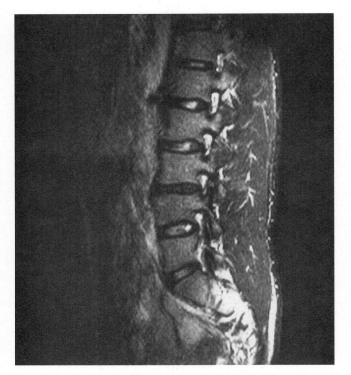

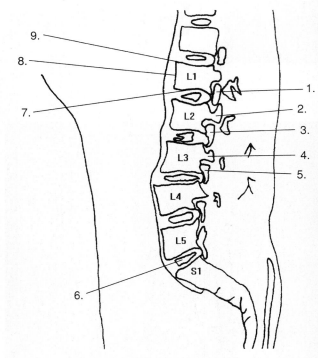

Figure 7-2

1. What number illustrates the superior vertebral
   endplate?
   _____ A. 1
   _____ B. 7
   _____ C. 2
   _____ D. 9

2. Which of the following is illustrated by 5?
   _____ A. L3 nerve roots
   _____ B. L2 nerve roots
   _____ C. L4 nerve roots
   _____ D. L3 pedicle

3. What number illustrates the L2 pedicle?
   _____ A. 4
   _____ B. 2
   _____ C. 5
   _____ D. 7

4. Which of the following is illustrated by 8?
   _____ A. Inferior vertebral endplate L1
   _____ B. L1 nerve roots
   _____ C. Anterior cortical bone of body
   _____ D. L2 nerve roots

5. Which of the following is illustrated by 6?
   _____ A. Anterior cortical bone of body
   _____ B. L3 pedicle
   _____ C. Intervertebral disk
   _____ D. Inferior vertebral endplate L1

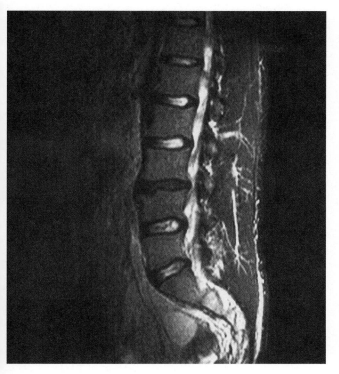
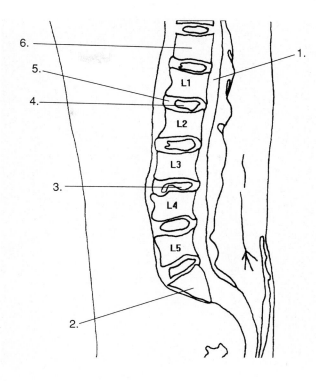

Figure 7-3

1. Which of the following is illustrated by 1?
   _____ A. Spinal cord
   _____ B. Edge of dural sac
   _____ C. Anulus fibrosus
   _____ D. Cauda equina

2. What number illustrates the herniated disk?
   _____ A. 4
   _____ B. 2
   _____ C. 5
   _____ D. 3

3. What number illustrates the nucleus pulposus?
   _____ A. 4
   _____ B. 6
   _____ C. 1
   _____ D. 5

4. Which of the following is illustrated by 6?
   _____ A. L1 vertebral body
   _____ B. L2 vertebral body
   _____ C. T12 vertebral body
   _____ D. Intervertebral disk

5. What number illustrates the anulus fibrosus?
   _____ A. 5
   _____ B. 1
   _____ C. 3
   _____ D. 4

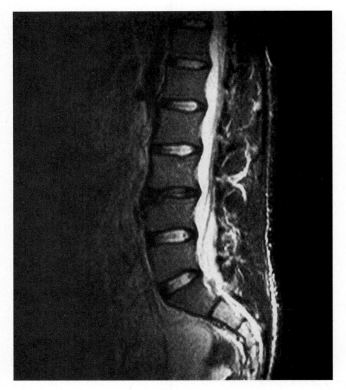
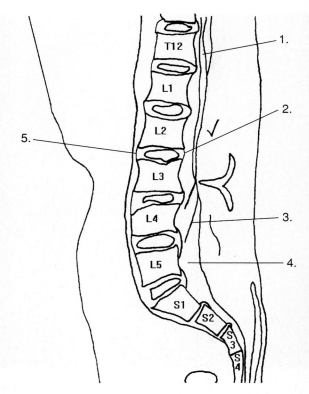

Figure 7-4

1. Which of the following is illustrated by 1?
   _____ A. Spinal cord
   _____ B. Edge of dural sac
   _____ C. Anulus fibrosus
   _____ D. Cauda equina

2. Which of the following is illustrated by 2?
   _____ A. Anterior longitudinal ligament
   _____ B. Posterior longitudinal ligament
   _____ C. Herniated disk
   _____ D. Nucleus pulposus

3. What number illustrates the cauda equina?
   _____ A. 1
   _____ B. 3
   _____ C. 4
   _____ D. 2

4. What number illustrates the subarachnoid space?
   _____ A. 1
   _____ B. 2
   _____ C. 3
   _____ D. 4

5. Which of the following is illustrated by 5?
   _____ A. Anterior longitudinal ligament
   _____ B. Posterior longitudinal ligament
   _____ C. Herniated disk
   _____ D. Nucleus pulposus

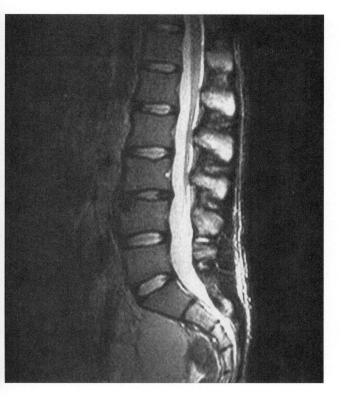
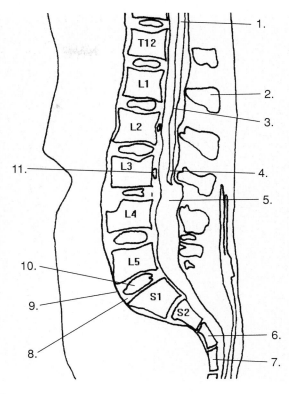

Figure 7-5

1. What number illustrates the conus medullaris?
  _____ A. 1
  _____ B. 5
  _____ C. 4
  _____ D. 3

2. Which of the following is illustrated by 10?
  _____ A. Intervertebral disk L4-L5
  _____ B. Nucleus pulposus
  _____ C. Anulus fibrosus
  _____ D. Intervertebral disk S1-S2

3. What number illustrates the spinal cord?
  _____ A. 5
  _____ B. 3
  _____ C. 1
  _____ D. 4

4. Which of the following is illustrated by 5?
  _____ A. Subarachnoid space
  _____ B. Epidural space
  _____ C. L1 spinous process
  _____ D. Subdural space

5. Which of the following is illustrated by 4?
  _____ A. Spinal cord
  _____ B. Conus medullaris
  _____ C. Cauda equina
  _____ D. Basivertebral vein

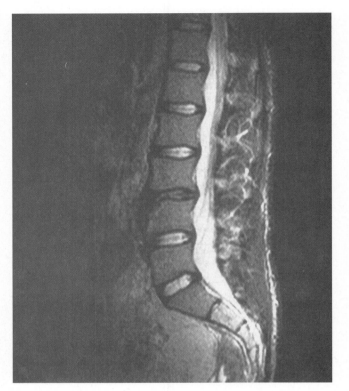

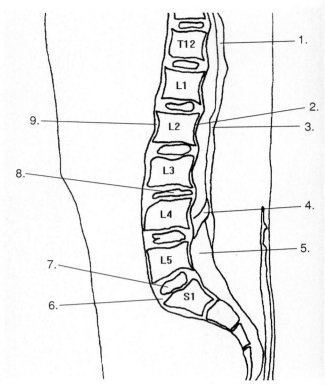

Figure 7-6

1. What number illustrates the cauda equina?
    _____ A. 1
    _____ B. 4
    _____ C. 3
    _____ D. 5

2. Which of the following is illustrated by 7?
    _____ A. Annulus fibrosus
    _____ B. Ruptured disk
    _____ C. Nucleus pulposus
    _____ D. Intervertebral disk L4-L5

3. Which of the following is illustrated by 2?
    _____ A. Anterior longitudinal ligament
    _____ B. Conus medullaris
    _____ C. Spinal cord
    _____ D. Posterior longitudinal ligament

4. Which of the following is illustrated by 9?
    _____ A. Anterior longitudinal ligament
    _____ B. Annulus fibrosus
    _____ C. Subarachnoid space
    _____ D. Posterior longitudinal ligament

5. What number illustrates the ruptured disk?
    _____ A. 7
    _____ B. 9
    _____ C. 5
    _____ D. 8

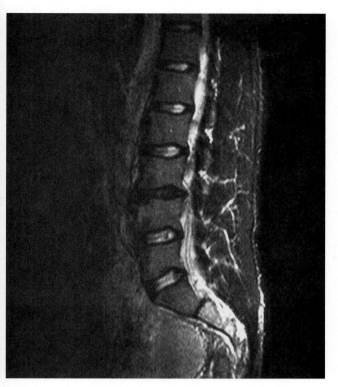
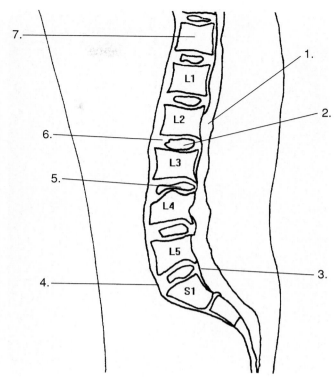

Figure 7-7

1. Which of the following is illustrated by 2?
   _____ A. Anulus fibrosus
   _____ B. Herniated disk
   _____ C. Nucleus pulposus
   _____ D. Edge of dural sac

2. What number illustrates the anterior longitudinal ligament?
   _____ A. 4
   _____ B. 3
   _____ C. 5
   _____ D. 2

3. Which of the following is illustrated by 6?
   _____ A. Herniated disk
   _____ B. Anulus fibrosus
   _____ C. Nucleus pulposus
   _____ D. Edge of dural sac

4. Which of the following is illustrated by 1?
   _____ A. Edge of the dural sac
   _____ B. Epidural space
   _____ C. Basivertebral vein
   _____ D. Pia mater

5. What number illustrates the herniated disk?
   _____ A. 2
   _____ B. 6
   _____ C. 4
   _____ D. 5

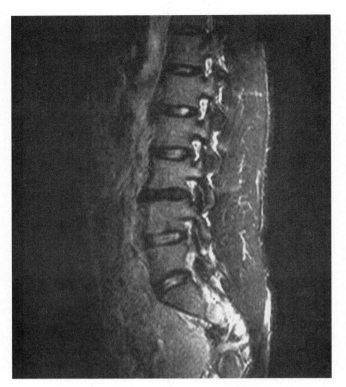
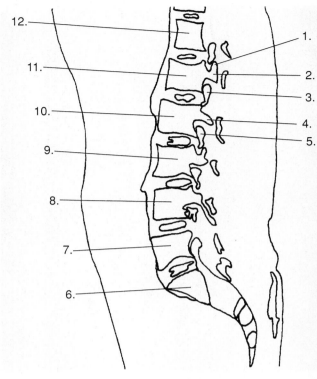

Figure 7-8

1. What number illustrates the L1 nerve roots?
   _____ A. 2
   _____ B. 5
   _____ C. 3
   _____ D. 1

2. Which of the following is illustrated by 10?
   _____ A. L2
   _____ B. L1
   _____ C. L3
   _____ D. T1

3. What number illustrates the L1 pedicle?
   _____ A. 4
   _____ B. 3
   _____ C. 5
   _____ D. 2

4. Which of the following is illustrated by 8?
   _____ A. L3
   _____ B. L4
   _____ C. S1
   _____ D. L5

5. Which of the following is illustrated by 3?
   _____ A. L2 nerve roots
   _____ B. L1 pedicle
   _____ C. L1 nerve roots
   _____ D. L2 pedicle

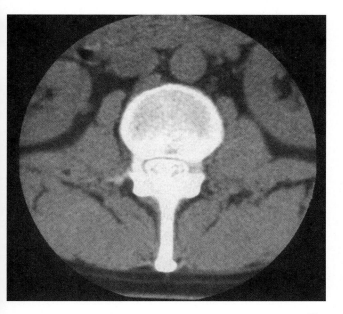 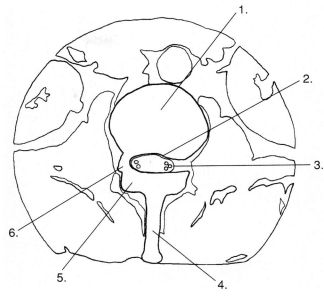

Figure 7-9

1. What number illustrates the epidural space?
   _____ A. 3
   _____ B. 2
   _____ C. 5
   _____ D. 6

2. Which of the following is illustrated by 4?
   _____ A. Lamina of L2
   _____ B. Pedicle of L2
   _____ C. L2 vertebral body
   _____ D. Spinous process of L2

3. What number illustrates the lamina of L2?
   _____ A. 5
   _____ B. 2
   _____ C. 6
   _____ D. 4

4. Which of the following is illustrated by 5?
   _____ A. Pedicle of L2
   _____ B. Lamina of L2
   _____ C. Spinous process of L2
   _____ D. Epidural space

5. Which of the following is illustrated by 3?
   _____ A. Spinal cord
   _____ B. Epidural space
   _____ C. Dural sac
   _____ D. Subarachnoid space

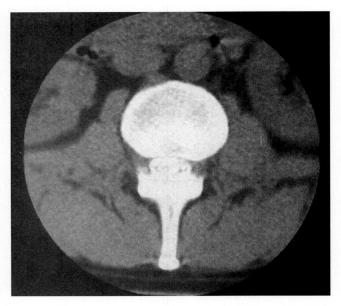
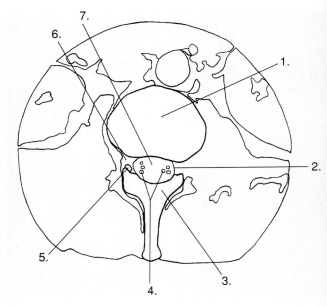

Figure 7-10

1. Which of the following is illustrated by 4?
   _____ A. Posterior dorsal root ganglion
   _____ B. Epidural space
   _____ C. Cauda equina
   _____ D. Conus medullaris

2. Which of the following is illustrated by 2?
   _____ A. Dural sac
   _____ B. Posterior dorsal root ganglion
   _____ C. Subarachnoid space
   _____ D. Cauda equina

3. Which of the following is illustrated by 6?
   _____ A. Vertebral foramen
   _____ B. Posterior (dorsal) root ganglion
   _____ C. Cauda equina
   _____ D. Intervertebral foramen

4. Which of the following is illustrated by 7?
   _____ A. Spinal cord
   _____ B. Subarachnoid space
   _____ C. Posterior dorsal root ganglion
   _____ D. Epidural space

5. Which of the following is illustrated by 5?
   _____ A. Cauda equina
   _____ B. Conus medullaris
   _____ C. Posterior (dorsal) root ganglion
   _____ D. Anterior nerve root

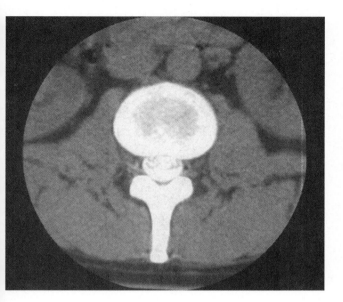 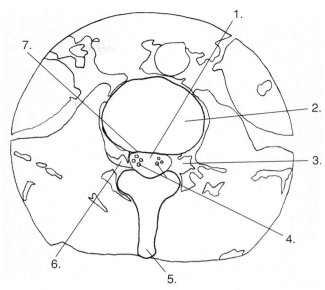

Figure 7-11

1. Which of the following is illustrated by 2?
   _____ A. Spinous process
   _____ B. Superior endplate
   _____ C. Inferior endplate
   _____ D. Intervertebral disk

2. What number illustrates the cauda equina?
   _____ A. 4
   _____ B. 7
   _____ C. 6
   _____ D. 1

3. Which of the following is illustrated by 7?
   _____ A. Pia mater
   _____ B. Arachnoid mater
   _____ C. Subarachnoid space
   _____ D. Dural sac

4. Which of the following is illustrated by 3?
   _____ A. Intervertebral disk
   _____ B. Intervertebral foramen
   _____ C. Dural sac
   _____ D. Cauda equina

5. What number illustrates the subarachnoid space?
   _____ A. 7
   _____ B. 4
   _____ C. 1
   _____ D. 6

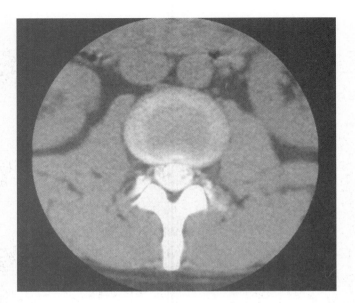 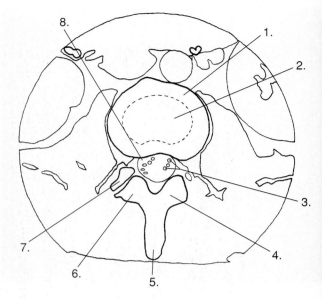

Figure 7-12

1. Which of the following is illustrated by 6?
   _____ A. Spinous process of L2
   _____ B. Lamina of L2
   _____ C. Superior articular process of L3
   _____ D. Inferior articular process of L2

2. What number illustrates the anulus fibrosus?
   _____ A. 8
   _____ B. 1
   _____ C. 4
   _____ D. 2

3. Which of the following is illustrated by 2?
   _____ A. Nucleus pulposus
   _____ B. Anulus fibrosus
   _____ C. Vertebral body of L3
   _____ D. Vertebral body of L2

4. What number illustrates the superior articular process of L3?
   _____ A. 5
   _____ B. 4
   _____ C. 7
   _____ D. 6

5. Which of the following is illustrated by 8?
   _____ A. Spinal cord
   _____ B. Subarachnoid space
   _____ C. Cauda equina
   _____ D. Conus medullaris

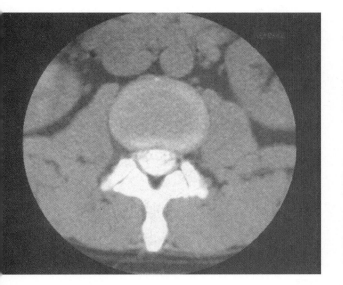
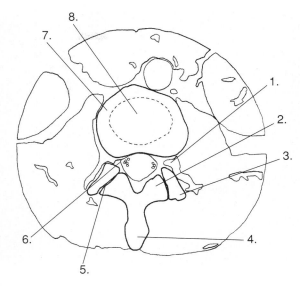

Figure 7-13

1. Which of the following is illustrated by 5?
   _____ A. Zygapophysis
   _____ B. Inferior articular process of L2
   _____ C. Lamina of L2
   _____ D. Epidural space

2. Which of the following is illustrated by 3?
   _____ A. Inferior articular process of L2
   _____ B. Lamina of L2
   _____ C. Superior articular process of L3
   _____ D. Pedicle of L2

3. What number illustrates the anulus fibrosus?
   _____ A. 8
   _____ B. 7
   _____ C. 6
   _____ D. 2

4. Which of the following is illustrated by 6?
   _____ A. Dural sac
   _____ B. Zygapophysis
   _____ C. Nucleus pulposus
   _____ D. Cauda equina

5. What number illustrates the inferior articular process of L2?
   _____ A. 1
   _____ B. 3
   _____ C. 6
   _____ D. 2

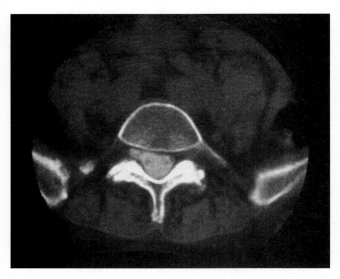

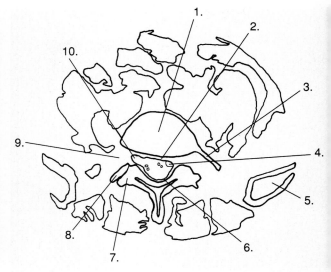

Figure 7-14

1. Which of the following is illustrated by 6?
   _____ A. Spinal cord
   _____ B. Dural sac
   _____ C. Conus medullaris
   _____ D. S1 nerve root

2. Which of the following is illustrated by 10?
   _____ A. Intervertebral foramen
   _____ B. Conus medullaris
   _____ C. Cauda equina
   _____ D. L5 nerve root

3. What number illustrates the epidural space?
   _____ A. 2
   _____ B. 7
   _____ C. 4
   _____ D. 9

4. Which of the following is illustrated by 9?
   _____ A. L5 nerve root
   _____ B. Posterior (dorsal) root ganglion
   _____ C. Intervertebral foramen
   _____ D. Dural sac

5. Which of the following is illustrated by 3?
   _____ A. Transverse process of L5
   _____ B. Lateral part of S1
   _____ C. Lamina of S1
   _____ D. Pedicle of S1

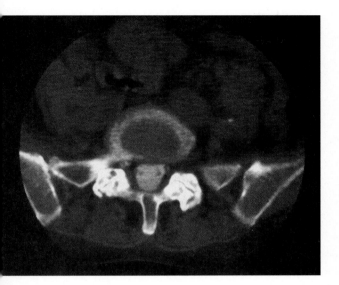
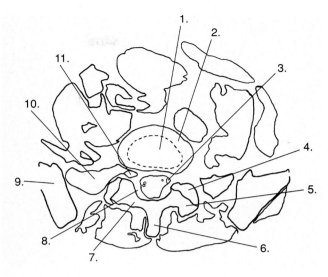

Figure 7-15

1. What number illustrates the lamina of L5?
   _____ A. 8
   _____ B. 7
   _____ C. 10
   _____ D. 5

2. Which of the following is illustrated by 3?
   _____ A. Spinal cord
   _____ B. Cauda equina
   _____ C. Epidural space
   _____ D. S1 nerve root

3. What number illustrates the nucleus pulposus?
   _____ A. 11
   _____ B. 8
   _____ C. 1
   _____ D. 2

4. What number illustrates the lateral part of S1?
   _____ A. 10
   _____ B. 4
   _____ C. 5
   _____ D. 9

5. Which of the following is illustrated by 5?
   _____ A. Superior articular process of S1
   _____ B. Superior articular process of L5
   _____ C. Inferior articular process of S1
   _____ D. Inferior articular process of L5

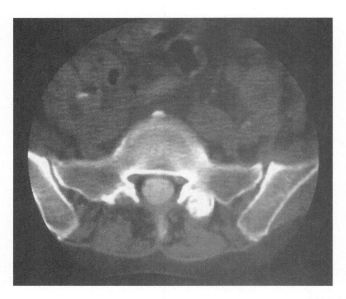
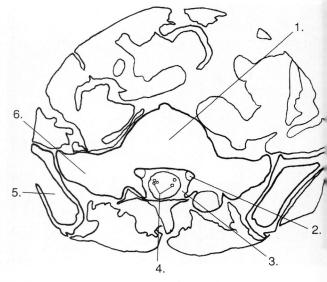

Figure 7-16

1. Which of the following is illustrated by 3?
   _____ A. S1 nerve root
   _____ B. Epidural space
   _____ C. Subarachnoid space
   _____ D. S2-S5 nerve roots

2. What number illustrates the ilium?
   _____ A. 6
   _____ B. 1
   _____ C. 2
   _____ D. 5

3. Which of the following is illustrated by 1?
   _____ A. Inferior endplate of L5
   _____ B. Intervertebral disk
   _____ C. Superior endplate of S1
   _____ D. Zygapophysis

4. Which of the following is illustrated by 6?
   _____ A. Lateral part of S1
   _____ B. Ilium
   _____ C. Transverse process of L5
   _____ D. Superior endplate of S1

5. Which of the following is illustrated by 4?
   _____ A. S1 nerve root
   _____ B. S2-S5 nerve roots
   _____ C. Dural sac
   _____ D. Epidural space

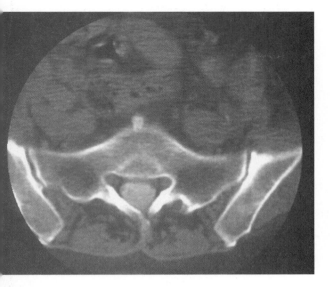 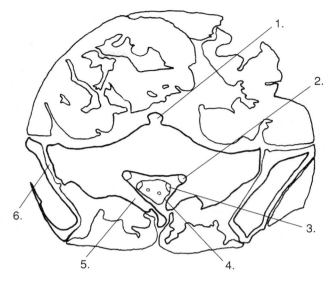

Figure 7-17

. What number illustrates the dural sac?

_____ A. 3
_____ B. 6
_____ C. 2
_____ D. 4

. Which of the following is illustrated by 2?

_____ A. S1 nerve root
_____ B. Subarachnoid space
_____ C. Vertebral artery
_____ D. Epidural space

. Which of the following is illustrated by 6?

_____ A. Lamina of S1
_____ B. Zygapophysis
_____ C. Sacroiliac joint
_____ D. L5-S1 intervertebral joint

4. What number illustrates the osteophyte?

_____ A. 5
_____ B. 1
_____ C. 6
_____ D. 2

5. Which of the following is illustrated by 3?

_____ A. Dural sac
_____ B. Epidural space
_____ C. Spinal cord
_____ D. S2 nerve root

CLINICAL APPLICATIONS

1. There are usually _____ cervical

   vertebrae, _____ thoracic

   vertebrae, _____ lumbar vertebrae,

   and _____ sacral segments.

2. The transverse foramina are characteristic of which of the following vertebrae?
   - _____ A. Cervical
   - _____ B. Lumbar
   - _____ C. Sacral
   - _____ D. Thoracic

3. Describe the posterior longitudinal ligament.

   _____

   _____

   _____

4. The anterior border of the right L5-S1 intervertebral

   foramen is formed by the_____,

   _____, and _____.

5. The conus medullaris is usually found at which of the following vertebral levels?
   - _____ A. T1-L2
   - _____ B. L1-L3
   - _____ C. L2-L4
   - _____ D. L3-L5

6. The _____ mater is the innermost meningeal layer.

7. In the spine, the upper and lower borders of the intervertebral foramen are formed by the
   - _____ A. Laminae
   - _____ B. Pedicles
   - _____ C. Articular processes
   - _____ D. Transverse processes

8. The [anterior/posterior] nerve root contains a collection of nerve cell bodies known as a ganglion.

   _____

   _____

   _____

9. In axial sections, which part of the vertebral column described as having a batlike appearance?

   _____

   _____

   _____

10. Which of the following have the largest vertebral foramina?
    - _____ A. Cervical
    - _____ B. Thoracic
    - _____ C. Lumbar
    - _____ D. Sacral

CLINICAL CORRELATIONS

■ Clinical Case 7-1

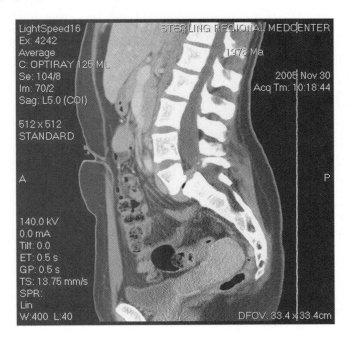

1. Which of the following best describes the image generated above?
   _____ A. T1 weighted magnetic resonance (MR)
   _____ B. T2 weighted MR
   _____ C. Computed tomography (CT)
   _____ D. Positron emission tomography (PET)/CT

2. In the image above, the injury is found at which of the following vertebral levels?
   _____ A. T12-L2
   _____ B. L1-L3
   _____ C. L3-L5
   _____ D. L5-S1

3. Which of the following best describes the injury?
   _____ A. Spondylolysis
   _____ B. Spondylolisthesis
   _____ C. Degenerative disk disease
   _____ D. Ankylosing spondylitis

4. Which of the following would most likely be affected by this injury?
   _____ A. Spinal cord
   _____ B. Cauda equina
   _____ C. Conus medullaris
   _____ D. Vagus nerve

5. Would the injury shown above result in a constriction of the spinal nerves?
   _____ A. Yes
   _____ B. No

■ Clinical Case 7-2

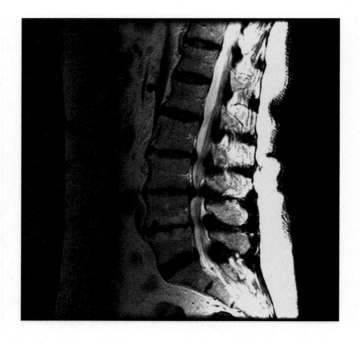

1. Which of the following best describes the image generated above?
   _____ A. T1 weighted magnetic resonance (MR)
   _____ B. T2 weighted MR
   _____ C. Computed tomography (CT)
   _____ D. Positron emission tomography (PET)/CT

2. In this image, does the spinal cord have a strong or weak signal?
   _____ A. Strong
   _____ B. Weak

3. Typically, the spinal cord terminates at what vertebral level?
   _____ A. T12-L2
   _____ B. L1-L3
   _____ C. L3-L5
   _____ D. L5-S1

4. The ventral nerve roots from the spinal cord transmit which of the following fibers?
   _____ A. Motor
   _____ B. Sensory
   _____ C. Both of the above
   _____ D. None of the above

5. In this image, does the cerebrospinal fluid have a strong or weak signal?
   _____ A. Strong
   _____ B. Weak

■ Clinical Case 7-3

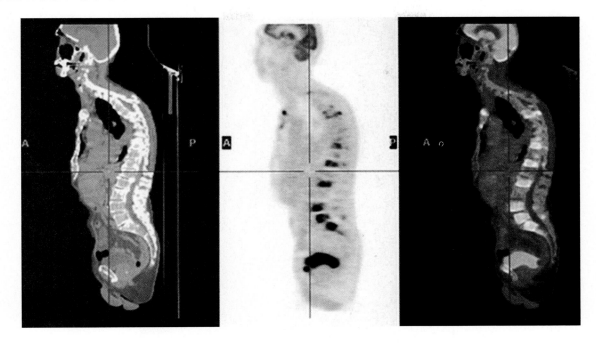

1. Describe the location of the metastatic disease within the spine on the CT (left), PET (middle), and corresponding fused PET/CT (right) images in this patient who was previously treated for adenocarcinoma of the colon.

   _____

   _____

   _____

2. Describe the changes in adjacent tissues.

   _____

   _____

   _____

3. Describe the consistency, shape, and border.

   _____

   _____

   _____

■ Clinical Case 7-4

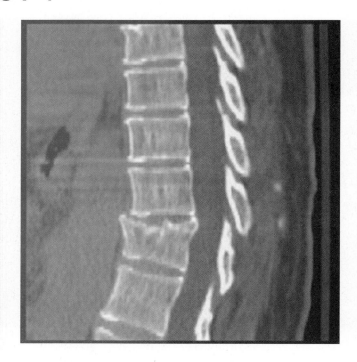

1. Describe the location of the pathology within the lower thoracic spine (T12 is lowest vertebra shown in full).

   _____

   _____

   _____

2. Describe the changes in adjacent tissues.

   _____

   _____

   _____

3. Describe the consistency, shape, and border.

   _____

   _____

   _____

Clinical Case 7-5

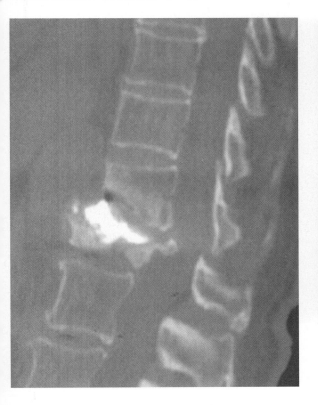
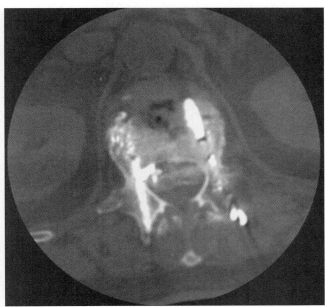

1. Describe the location of the pathology within the spine in this patient who previously underwent vertebroplasty (the upper part of L3 is the lowermost vertebra shown).

_____

_____

_____

2. Describe the changes in adjacent tissues.

_____

_____

_____

3. Describe the consistency, shape, and border.

_____

_____

_____

■ Clinical Case 7-6

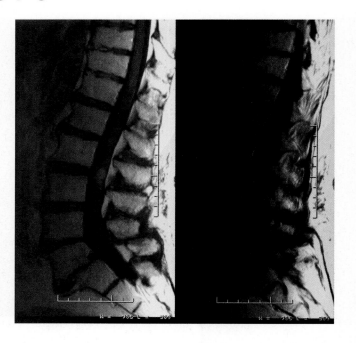

1. Describe the location of the metastatic disease shown in this MR imaging examination following the administration of 15 cc of gadolinium.

   _____

   _____

   _____

2. Describe the changes in adjacent tissues.

   _____

   _____

   _____

3. Describe the consistency, shape, and border.

   _____

   _____

   _____

■ Clinical Case 7-7

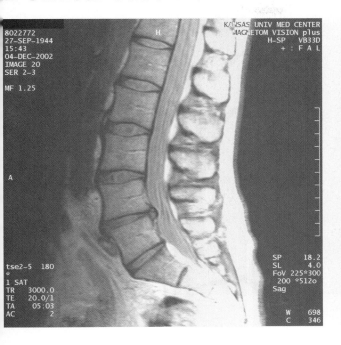

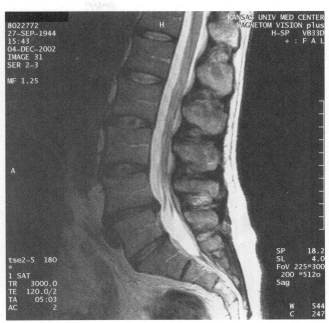

1. Describe the location of the pathology shown with proton density (left) and T2 (right) weighted MR sagittal images in the spine of this 58-year-old patient reporting chronic lower back pain.

_____

_____

_____

2. Describe the changes in adjacent tissues.

_____

_____

_____

3. Describe the consistency, shape, and border.

_____

_____

_____

■ Clinical Case 7-8

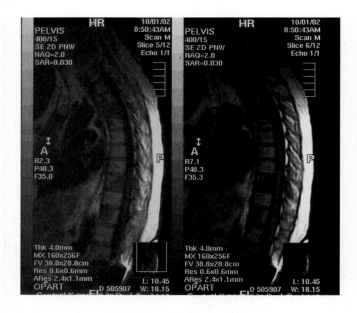

1. Describe the location of the pathology shown with T1 weighted MR sagittal images in the spine of this female patient previously treated for malignant breast carcinoma (T12 is lowest vertebra shown completely).

   _____

   _____

   _____

2. Describe the changes in adjacent tissues.

   _____

   _____

   _____

3. Describe the consistency, shape, and border.

   _____

   _____

   _____

Chapter 8

Joints

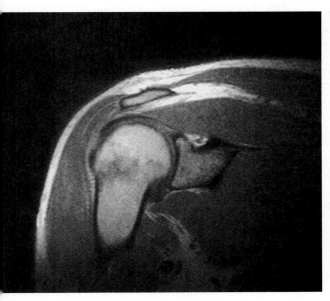

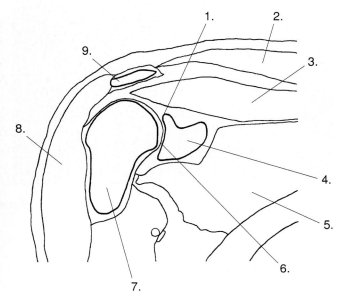

Figure 8-1

1. Which of the following illustrates 6?
   _____ A. Glenohumeral joint
   _____ B. Acromioclavicular joint
   _____ C. Axillary recess
   _____ D. Inferior glenoid labrum

2. Which number illustrates the trapezius muscle?
   _____ A. 3
   _____ B. 2
   _____ C. 5
   _____ D. 8

3. Which of the following is illustrated by 4?
   _____ A. Superior glenoid labrum
   _____ B. Glenohumeral joint
   _____ C. Acromion process of scapula
   _____ D. Glenoid process of scapula

4. Which of the following is illustrated by 1?
   _____ A. Superior glenoid labrum
   _____ B. Acromion process
   _____ C. Axillary recess
   _____ D. Acromioclavicular joint

5. Which number illustrates the supraspinatus muscle?
   _____ A. 2
   _____ B. 5
   _____ C. 3
   _____ D. 8

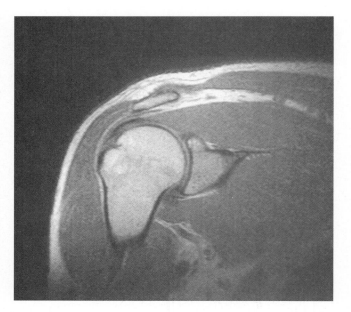
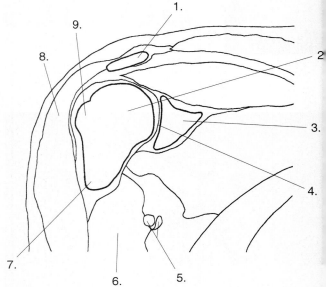

Figure 8-2

1. Which of the following is illustrated by 6?
   _____ A. Subscapular muscle
   _____ B. Teres minor muscle
   _____ C. Deltoid muscle
   _____ D. Teres major muscle

2. Which of the following is illustrated by 9?
   _____ A. Lesser tubercle of the humerus
   _____ B. Greater tubercle of the humerus
   _____ C. Surgical neck
   _____ D. Head of the humerus

3. Which of the following is illustrated by 1?
   _____ A. Greater tubercle of the humerus
   _____ B. Surgical neck of the humerus
   _____ C. Acromion process of the scapula
   _____ D. Head of the humerus

4. Which of the following is illustrated by 7?
   _____ A. Surgical neck of the humerus
   _____ B. Greater tubercle of the humerus
   _____ C. Head of the humerus
   _____ D. Acromion process of the scapula

5. Which of the following is illustrated by 2?
   _____ A. Acromion process of the scapula
   _____ B. Greater tubercle of the humerus
   _____ C. Head of the humerus
   _____ D. Surgical neck of the humerus

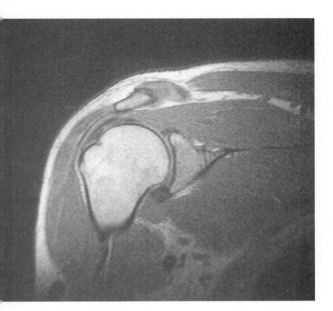
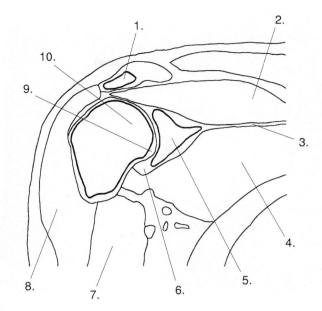

Figure 8-3

. Which of the following is illustrated by 1?
_____ A. Glenoid process of scapula
_____ B. Clavicle
_____ C. Greater tubercle
_____ D. Acromion process of scapula

. Which number illustrates the supraspinatus muscle?
_____ A. 2
_____ B. 8
_____ C. 7
_____ D. 4

. Which of the following is illustrated by 6?
_____ A. Axillary recess of the articular cavity
_____ B. Glenoid process of the scapula
_____ C. Acromioclavicular joint
_____ D. Articular cartilage

4. Which number illustrates the articular cartilage?
_____ A. 3
_____ B. 10
_____ C. 9
_____ D. 6

5. Which of the following is illustrated by 3?
_____ A. Articular cartilage
_____ B. Glenoid labrum
_____ C. Glenoid process of scapula
_____ D. Body of scapula

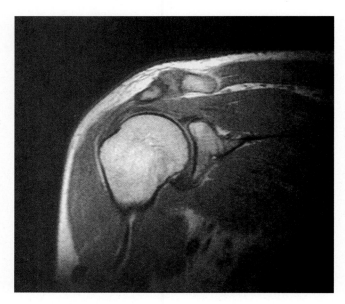
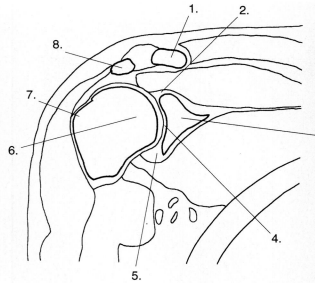

Figure 8-4

1. Which of the following is illustrated by 2?
   _____ A. Articular cartilage in the glenoid fossa
   _____ B. Superior glenoid labrum
   _____ C. Inferior glenoid labrum
   _____ D. Axillary recess of articular cavity

2. Which of the following is illustrated by 1?
   _____ A. Acromion process of scapula
   _____ B. Glenoid process of scapula
   _____ C. Superior glenoid labrum
   _____ D. Clavicle

3. Which number illustrates the articular cartilage in the glenoid fossa?
   _____ A. 4
   _____ B. 3
   _____ C. 2
   _____ D. 5

4. Which number illustrates the inferior glenoid labrum?
   _____ A. 4
   _____ B. 3
   _____ C. 5
   _____ D. 2

5. Which of the following is illustrated by 3?
   _____ A. Superior glenoid labrum
   _____ B. Inferior glenoid labrum
   _____ C. Glenoid process of the scapula
   _____ D. Acromion process of the scapula

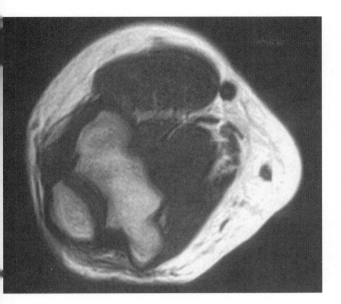

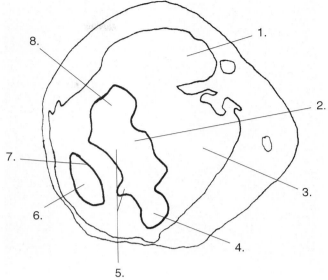

Figure 8-5

1. Which illustrates the trochlear notch?
   _____ A. 4
   _____ B. 7
   _____ C. 6
   _____ D. 5

2. Which of the following is illustrated by 2?
   _____ A. Radius
   _____ B. Ulna
   _____ C. Trochlea
   _____ D. Humerus

3. Which number illustrates the olecranon process of the ulna?
   _____ A. 7
   _____ B. 2
   _____ C. 6
   _____ D. 5

4. Which of the following is illustrated by 4?
   _____ A. Medial epicondyle
   _____ B. Capitulum
   _____ C. Trochlea
   _____ D. Lateral epicondyle

5. Which of the following is illustrated by 1?
   _____ A. Biceps muscle
   _____ B. Triceps muscle
   _____ C. Brachialis muscle
   _____ D. Brachioradialis muscle

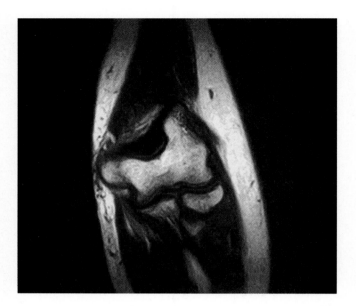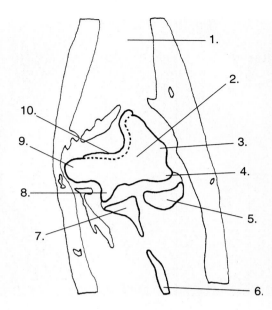

Figure 8-6

1. Which of the following is illustrated by 8?
   _____ A. Coronoid process of ulna
   _____ B. Medial epicondyle
   _____ C. Trochlea
   _____ D. Capitulum

2. Which number illustrates the capitulum?
   _____ A. 4
   _____ B. 2
   _____ C. 5
   _____ D. 3

3. Which of the following is illustrated by 10?
   _____ A. Capitulum
   _____ B. Lateral epicondyle
   _____ C. Trochlea
   _____ D. Olecranon fossa

4. Which number illustrates the lateral epicondyle?
   _____ A. 7
   _____ B. 3
   _____ C. 5
   _____ D. 9

5. Which number illustrates the coronoid process of the ulna?
   _____ A. 5
   _____ B. 6
   _____ C. 9
   _____ D. 7

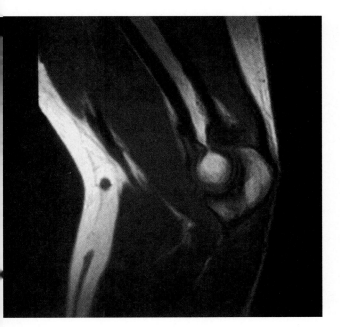

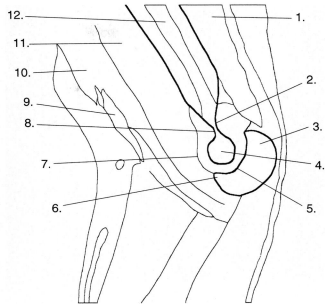

Figure 8-7

1. Which number illustrates the olecranon fossa?
   _____ A. 8
   _____ B. 5
   _____ C. 7
   _____ D. 2

2. Which of the following is illustrated by 5?
   _____ A. Olecranon process of ulna
   _____ B. Articular capsule
   _____ C. Trochlear notch
   _____ D. Coronoid process of ulna

3. Which number illustrates the triceps muscle?
   _____ A. 1
   _____ B. 12
   _____ C. 11
   _____ D. 10

4. Which of the following is illustrated by 9?
   _____ A. Brachialis muscle
   _____ B. Brachial artery
   _____ C. Biceps muscle
   _____ D. Axillary artery

5. Which of the following is illustrated by 7?
   _____ A. Capitulum
   _____ B. Coronoid fossa
   _____ C. Articular capsule
   _____ D. Trochlear notch

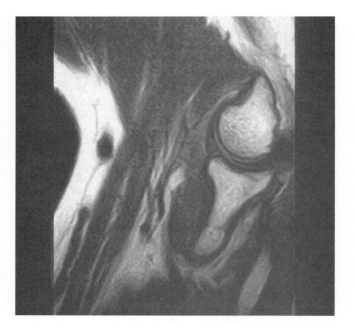

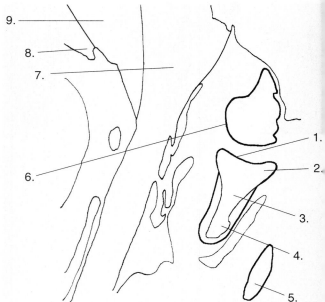

Figure 8-8

1. Which of the following is illustrated by 3?
   _____ A. Fovea of the radius
   _____ B. Neck of radius
   _____ C. Radial tuberosity
   _____ D. Head of radius

2. Which number illustrates the biceps muscle?
   _____ A. 8
   _____ B. 6
   _____ C. 9
   _____ D. 7

3. Which of the following is illustrated by 7?
   _____ A. Biceps muscle
   _____ B. Deltoid muscle
   _____ C. Brachialis muscle
   _____ D. Brachioradialis muscle

4. Which number illustrates the fovea of the radius?
   _____ A. 2
   _____ B. 5
   _____ C. 1
   _____ D. 6

5. Which number illustrates the capitulum?
   _____ A. 6
   _____ B. 2
   _____ C. 1
   _____ D. 5

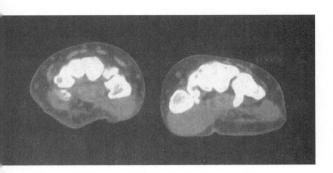
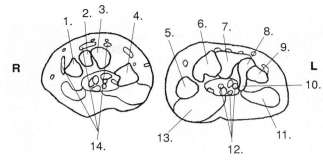

Figure 8-9

. Which of the following is illustrated by 9?
_____ A. Trapezoid
_____ B. Triquetrum
_____ C. Trapezium
_____ D. Hamate

. Which number illustrates the trapezoid?
_____ A. 4
_____ B. 2
_____ C. 7
_____ D. 3

. Which of the following is illustrated by 6?
_____ A. Trapezium
_____ B. Hamate
_____ C. Trapezoid
_____ D. Capitate

4. Which number illustrates the abductor digiti minimi muscle?
_____ A. 11
_____ B. 13
_____ C. 12
_____ D. 14

5. Which number illustrates the flexor digitorum superficialis and profundus tendons?
_____ A. 14
_____ B. 13
_____ C. 11
_____ D. 12

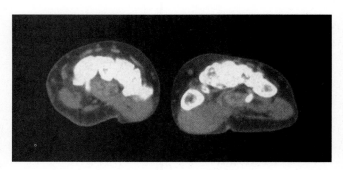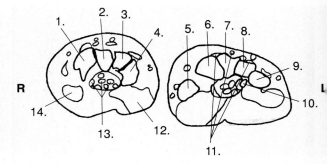

Figure 8-10

1. Which number illustrates the capitate?
   _____ A. 8
   _____ B. 6
   _____ C. 3
   _____ D. 7

2. Which of the following is illustrated by 10?
   _____ A. Triquetrum
   _____ B. Hamulus of hamate
   _____ C. Pisiform
   _____ D. Scaphoid

3. Which number illustrates the right hamate?
   _____ A. 3
   _____ B. 1
   _____ C. 4
   _____ D. 2

4. Which of the following is illustrated by 11?
   _____ A. Extensor tendons
   _____ B. Flexor digitorum superficialis and profundus
         tendons
   _____ C. Abductor digiti minimi muscle
   _____ D. Abductor pollicis brevis and opponens
         pollicis muscles

5. Which of the following is illustrated by 13?
   _____ A. Extensor tendons
   _____ B. Flexor digitorum superficialis and profundus
         tendons
   _____ C. Abductor digiti minimi muscle
   _____ D. Abductor pollicis brevis and opponens
         pollicis muscles

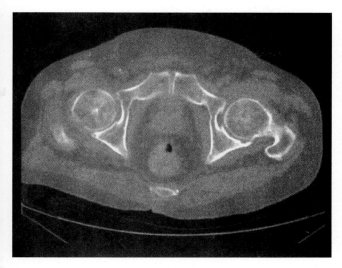
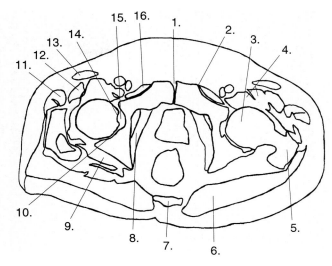

Figure 8-11

1. Which number illustrates the sartorius muscle?
   _____ A. 14
   _____ B. 13
   _____ C. 12
   _____ D. 11

2. Which of the following is illustrated by 14?
   _____ A. Acetabular fossa
   _____ B. Lunate surface of acetabulum
   _____ C. Fovea capitis femoris
   _____ D. Pubic symphysis

3. Which number illustrates the tensor fascia latae muscle?
   _____ A. 11
   _____ B. 14
   _____ C. 12
   _____ D. 13

4. Which of the following is illustrated by 1?
   _____ A. Pubic symphysis
   _____ B. Acetabular fossa
   _____ C. Obturator foramen
   _____ D. Sacroiliac joint

5. Which number illustrates the superior gemellus muscle?
   _____ A. 9
   _____ B. 8
   _____ C. 6
   _____ D. 4

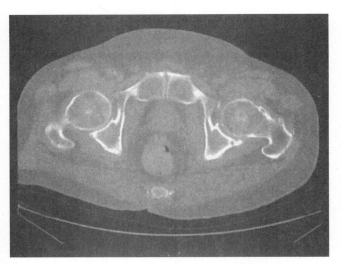
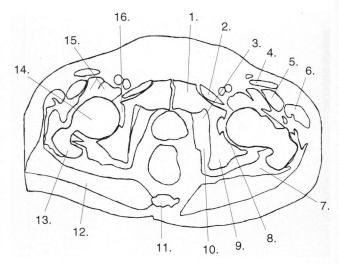

Figure 8-12

1. Which of the following is illustrated by 3?
   _____ A. Lunate surface of acetabulum
   _____ B. Obturator foramen
   _____ C. Pubic symphysis
   _____ D. Acetabular fossa

2. Which of the following is illustrated by 16?
   _____ A. Obturator foramen
   _____ B. Lunate surface of acetabulum
   _____ C. Fovea capitis femoris
   _____ D. Acetabular fossa

3. Which number illustrates the iliopsoas muscle?
   _____ A. 5
   _____ B. 10
   _____ C. 7
   _____ D. 15

4. Which number illustrates the obturator internus muscle?
   _____ A. 10
   _____ B. 15
   _____ C. 7
   _____ D. 2

5. Which illustrates the pectineus muscle?
   _____ A. 10
   _____ B. 15
   _____ C. 7
   _____ D. 2

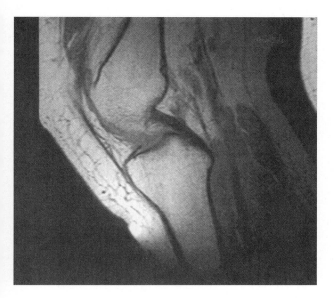
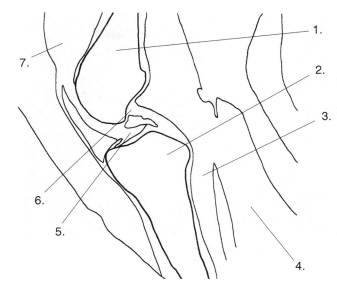

Figure 8-13

1. Which of the following is illustrated by 6?
_____ A. Posterior cruciate ligament
_____ B. Popliteus muscle
_____ C. Anterior cruciate ligament
_____ D. Tibia

2. Which of the following is illustrated by 2?
_____ A. Femur
_____ B. Fibula
_____ C. Patella
_____ D. Tibia

3. Which number illustrates the popliteus muscle?
_____ A. 4
_____ B. 7
_____ C. 5
_____ D. 3

4. Which of the following is illustrated by 5?
_____ A. Medial collateral ligament
_____ B. Anterior cruciate ligament
_____ C. Posterior cruciate ligament
_____ D. Popliteus muscle

5. Which number illustrates the quadriceps muscle?
_____ A. 7
_____ B. 4
_____ C. 6
_____ D. 3

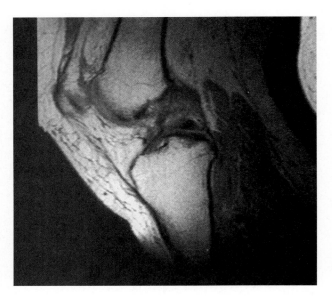
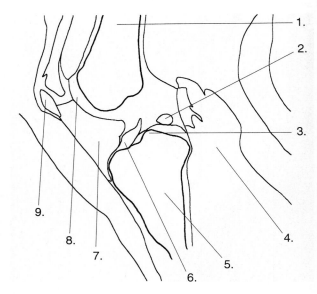

Figure 8-14

1. Which of the following is illustrated by 9?
    _____ A. Articular cartilage
    _____ B. Infrapatellar fat pad
    _____ C. Anterior cruciate ligament
    _____ D. Medial patella

2. Which of the following is illustrated by 3?
    _____ A. Posterior cruciate ligament
    _____ B. Intercondylar eminence
    _____ C. Anterior cruciate ligament
    _____ D. Lateral head of gastrocnemius muscle

3. Which number illustrates the anterior cruciate ligament?
    _____ A. 6
    _____ B. 8
    _____ C. 3
    _____ D. 2

4. Which of the following is illustrated by 7?
    _____ A. Patellar tendon
    _____ B. Patella
    _____ C. Infrapatellar fat pad
    _____ D. Quadriceps tendon

5. Which number illustrates the articular cartilage?
    _____ A. 8
    _____ B. 3
    _____ C. 2
    _____ D. 6

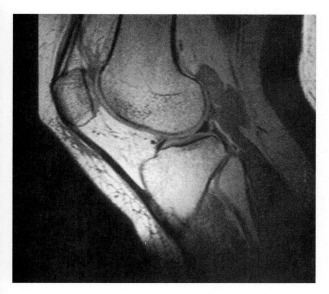
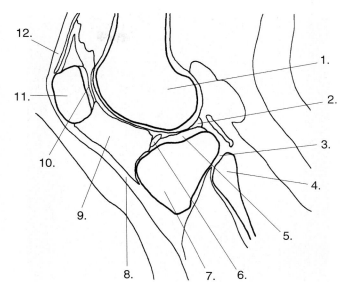

Figure 8-15

1. Which number illustrates the posterior horn of the lateral meniscus?
   _____ A. 5
   _____ B. 2
   _____ C. 7
   _____ D. 6

2. Which number illustrates the femoropatellar joint?
   _____ A. 5
   _____ B. 3
   _____ C. 9
   _____ D. 10

3. Which of the following is illustrated by 5?
   _____ A. Head of fibula
   _____ B. Anterior horn of lateral meniscus
   _____ C. Posterior horn of lateral meniscus
   _____ D. Articular cartilage

4. Which number illustrates the patella?
   _____ A. 11
   _____ B. 8
   _____ C. 9
   _____ D. 1

5. Which of the following is illustrated by 6?
   _____ A. Anterior horn of medial meniscus
   _____ B. Anterior cruciate ligament
   _____ C. Posterior cruciate ligament
   _____ D. Anterior horn of lateral meniscus

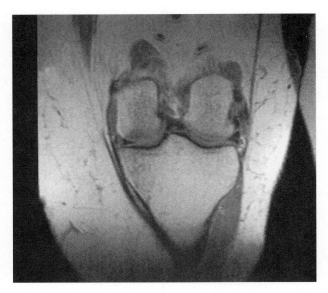

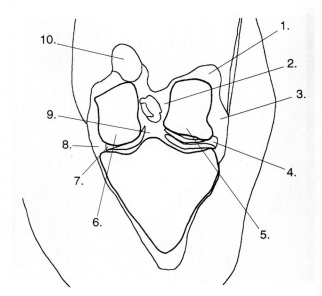

Figure 8-16

1. Which of the following is illustrated by 4?
   _____ A. Posterior cruciate ligament
   _____ B. Lateral collateral ligament
   _____ C. Lateral meniscus
   _____ D. Articular cartilage

2. Which number illustrates the posterior cruciate ligament?
   _____ A. 6
   _____ B. 2
   _____ C. 5
   _____ D. 9

3. Which number illustrates the medial meniscus?
   _____ A. 7
   _____ B. 9
   _____ C. 8
   _____ D. 4

4. Which of the following is illustrated by 1?
   _____ A. Lateral head of gastrocnemius muscle
   _____ B. Popliteal tendon
   _____ C. Quadriceps muscle
   _____ D. Medial head of gastrocnemius muscle

5. Which of the following is illustrated by 2?
   _____ A. Lateral collateral ligament
   _____ B. Anterior cruciate ligament
   _____ C. Medial meniscus
   _____ D. Posterior cruciate ligament

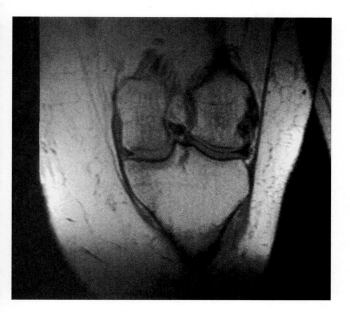
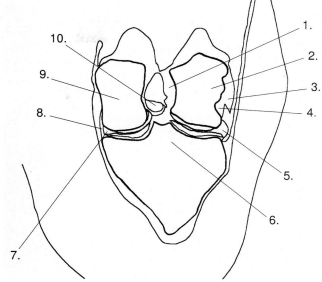

Figure 8-17

1. Which of the following is illustrated by 4?
   _____ A. Lateral collateral ligament
   _____ B. Lateral meniscus
   _____ C. Lateral epicondyle
   _____ D. Popliteal tendon

2. Which number illustrates the medial meniscus?
   _____ A. 7
   _____ B. 5
   _____ C. 8
   _____ D. 10

3. Which of the following is illustrated by 10?
   _____ A. Lateral meniscus
   _____ B. Posterior cruciate ligament
   _____ C. Medial meniscus
   _____ D. Anterior cruciate ligament

4. Which number illustrates the tibial intercondylar eminence?
   _____ A. 6
   _____ B. 10
   _____ C. 8
   _____ D. 5

5. Which of the following is illustrated by 2?
   _____ A. Lateral femoral epicondyle
   _____ B. Lateral femoral condyle
   _____ C. Head of fibula
   _____ D. Proximal tibia

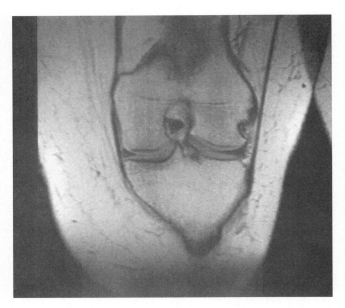

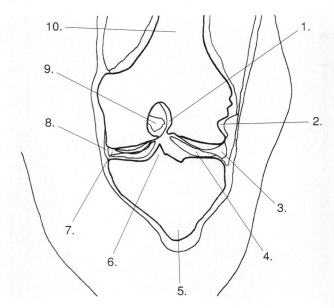

Figure 8-18

1. Which number illustrates the medial collateral ligament?
   _____ A. 8
   _____ B. 7
   _____ C. 4
   _____ D. 9

2. Which of the following is illustrated by 6?
   _____ A. Articular surface of tibia
   _____ B. Intercondylar eminence
   _____ C. Medial meniscus
   _____ D. Lateral meniscus

3. Which of the following is illustrated by 9?
   _____ A. Anterior cruciate ligament
   _____ B. Intercondylar eminence
   _____ C. Posterior cruciate ligament
   _____ D. Medial collateral ligament

4. Which number illustrates the popliteal tendon?
   _____ A. 1
   _____ B. 9
   _____ C. 3
   _____ D. 2

5. Which of the following is illustrated by 4?
   _____ A. Articular surface of tibia
   _____ B. Intercondylar eminence
   _____ C. Medial meniscus
   _____ D. Lateral meniscus

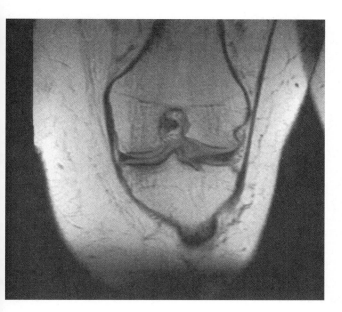
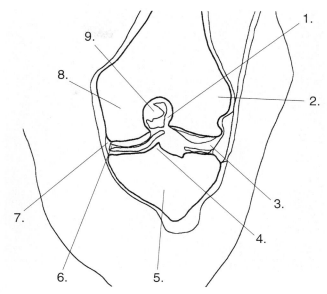

Figure 8-19

1. Which number illustrates the posterior cruciate
   ligament?
   _____ A. 1
   _____ B. 9
   _____ C. 4
   _____ D. 3

2. Which of the following is illustrated by 7?
   _____ A. Medial meniscus
   _____ B. Intercondylar eminence
   _____ C. Medial collateral ligament
   _____ D. Lateral meniscus

3. Which number illustrates the anterior cruciate
   ligament?
   _____ A. 1
   _____ B. 8
   _____ C. 2
   _____ D. 9

4. Which of the following is illustrated by 3?
   _____ A. Articular surface of medial condyle
   _____ B. Articular surface of tibia
   _____ C. Anterior cruciate ligament
   _____ D. Lateral meniscus

5. Which number illustrates the medial meniscus?
   _____ A. 6
   _____ B. 7
   _____ C. 3
   _____ D. 9

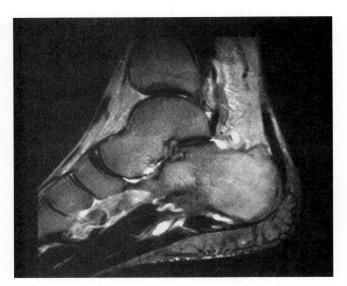 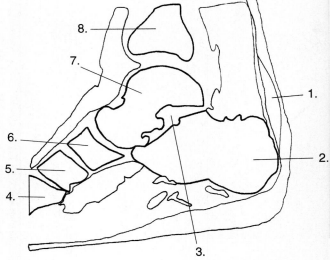

Figure 8-20

1. Which of the following is illustrated by 4?
   _____ A. First cuneiform
   _____ B. Navicular
   _____ C. First metatarsal
   _____ D. First digit

2. Which number illustrates the tibia?
   _____ A. 1
   _____ B. 8
   _____ C. 3
   _____ D. 7

3. Which of the following is illustrated by 7?
   _____ A. Navicular bone
   _____ B. Calcaneus
   _____ C. Tibia
   _____ D. Talus

4. Which number illustrates the tendinous insertion of gastrocnemius muscles?
   _____ A. 1
   _____ B. 3
   _____ C. 6
   _____ D. 2

5. Which of the following is illustrated by 5?
   _____ A. First cuneiform
   _____ B. Talus
   _____ C. Navicular
   _____ D. First metatarsal

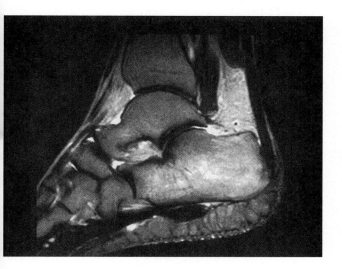

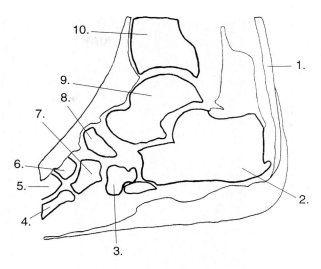

Figure 8-21

1. Which of the following is illustrated by 6?
   _____ A. Third metatarsal
   _____ B. Second metatarsal
   _____ C. Third cuneiform
   _____ D. Second cuneiform

2. Which number illustrates the talus?
   _____ A. 7
   _____ B. 9
   _____ C. 8
   _____ D. 2

3. Which number illustrates the third cuneiform?
   _____ A. 6
   _____ B. 4
   _____ C. 7
   _____ D. 5

4. Which of the following is illustrated by 2?
   _____ A. Calcaneus
   _____ B. Talus
   _____ C. Tibia
   _____ D. Tendo calcaneus tendon

5. Which of the following is illustrated by 8?
   _____ A. Cuboid
   _____ B. Navicular
   _____ C. Talus
   _____ D. Second cuneiform

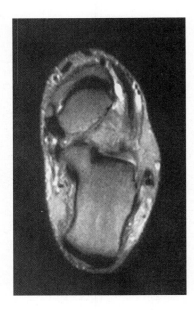

M 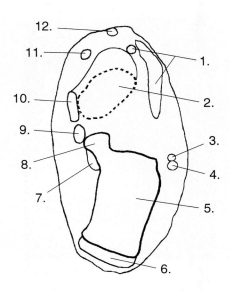 L

Figure 8-22

1. Which number illustrates the tibialis anterior tendon?
   _____ A. 1
   _____ B. 11
   _____ C. 9
   _____ D. 12

2. Which of the following is illustrated by 8?
   _____ A. Cuboid
   _____ B. Talus
   _____ C. Navicular
   _____ D. Sustentaculum tali

3. Which of the following is illustrated by 3?
   _____ A. Peroneus longus tendon
   _____ B. Flexor hallucis longus tendon
   _____ C. Flexor digitorum longus tendon
   _____ D. Peroneus brevis tendon

4. Which number illustrates the extensor digitorum tendon?
   _____ A. 1
   _____ B. 11
   _____ C. 4
   _____ D. 10

5. Which number illustrates the extensor hallucis longus tendon?
   _____ A. 11
   _____ B. 1
   _____ C. 12
   _____ D. 10

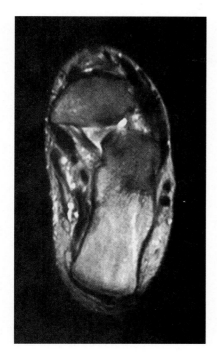

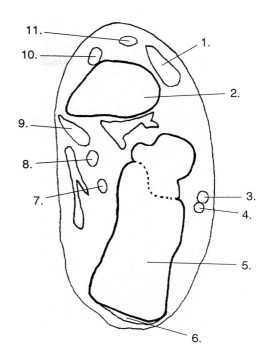

M   L

Figure 8-23

1. Which number illustrates the tibialis posterior tendon?
   _____ A. 10
   _____ B. 3
   _____ C. 9
   _____ D. 7

2. Which of the following is illustrated by 10?
   _____ A. Extensor hallucis longus tendon
   _____ B. Tibialis anterior tendon
   _____ C. Extensor digitorum tendon
   _____ D. Tibialis posterior tendon

3. Which number illustrates the peroneus brevis tendon?
   _____ A. 3
   _____ B. 7
   _____ C. 4
   _____ D. 8

4. Which of the following is illustrated by 5?
   _____ A. Cuboid
   _____ B. Talus
   _____ C. Sustentaculum tali
   _____ D. Calcaneus

5. Which number illustrates the talus?
   _____ A. 2
   _____ B. 5
   _____ C. 1
   _____ D. 9

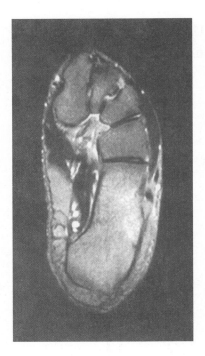

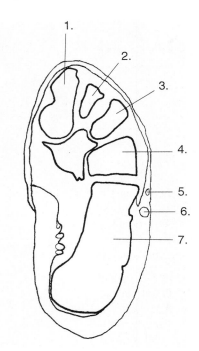

Figure 8-24

1. Which of the following is illustrated by 4?
   _____ A. Cuboid
   _____ B. Third cuneiform
   _____ C. Second cuneiform
   _____ D. Navicular

2. Which number illustrates the third cuneiform?
   _____ A. 2
   _____ B. 7
   _____ C. 4
   _____ D. 8

3. Which number illustrates the second cuneiform?
   _____ A. 3
   _____ B. 2
   _____ C. 4
   _____ D. 1

4. Which of the following is illustrated by 5?
   _____ A. Peroneus longus tendon
   _____ B. Extensor digitorum tendon
   _____ C. Peroneus brevis tendon
   _____ D. Extensor hallucis longus tendon

5. Which of the following is illustrated by 1?
   _____ A. Second cuneiform
   _____ B. Third cuneiform
   _____ C. First cuneiform
   _____ D. Cuboid

CLINICAL APPLICATIONS

----

1. The ankle joint is formed between the

   _____,

   _____, and

   _____.

2. The ankle joint is classified as what type of joint?
   _____ A. Ginglymus
   _____ B. Arthrodial
   _____ C. Enarthrosis
   _____ D. Syndesmosis

3. The hip joint is classified as what type of joint?
   _____ A. Ginglymus
   _____ B. Arthrodial
   _____ C. Enarthrosis
   _____ D. Syndesmosis

4. The _____ joint is considered the largest joint in the body.

5. Which of the following articulates with the base of the third metatarsal?
   _____ A. Cuboid
   _____ B. Navicular
   _____ C. Second cuneiform
   _____ D. Third cuneiform

6. Describe the attachments of the lateral collateral ligament.

   _____

   _____

   _____

7. The trochlea of the humerus articulates with the
   _____ A. Glenoid fossa
   _____ B. Clavicle
   _____ C. Radius
   _____ D. Ulna

8. On an axial image of the ankle, which tendon is *not* found on the medial surface of the leg?
   _____ A. Peroneus longus
   _____ B. Tibialis posterior
   _____ C. Flexor hallucis longus
   _____ D. Flexor digitorum longus

9. Approximately 75% of carpal fractures are found

   within the _____.

10. The hamulus is found on which carpal bone?
    _____ A. Scaphoid
    _____ B. Hamate
    _____ C. Capitate
    _____ D. Lunate

CLINICAL CORRELATIONS

■ Clinical Case 8-1

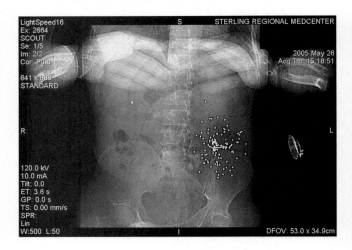

1. Which of the following is the correct classification for the hip joint?
   _____ A. Enarthrosis
   _____ B. Arthrodial
   _____ C. Syndesmosis
   _____ D. Ginglymus

2. Which of the following bones form the acetabulum?
   _____ A. Pubis
   _____ B. Ischium
   _____ C. Ilium
   _____ D. All of the above

3. Which of the following best describes the location of the tensor fascia latae muscle as compared to the hip joint?
   _____ A. Medial
   _____ B. Lateral
   _____ C. Anterior
   _____ D. Posterior

4. What muscle originates from the ischial spine and inserts on the tendon of the obturator internus muscle rotating the thigh laterally?
   _____ A. Sartorius
   _____ B. Rectus femoris
   _____ C. Superior gemellus
   _____ D. Pectineus

5. What muscle originates from the pubis to insert on the femur and also acts to rotate the thigh laterally?
   _____ A. Sartorius
   _____ B. Rectus femoris
   _____ C. Superior gemellus
   _____ D. Pectineus

■ Clinical Case 8-2

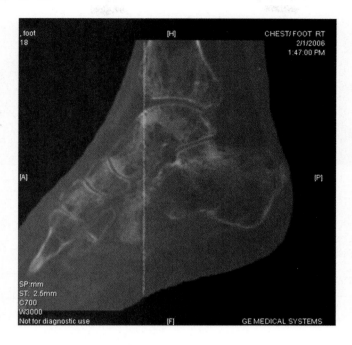

1. Which of the following best describes the condition shown above?
   - _____ A. Osteopetrosis
   - _____ B. Osteoporosis
   - _____ C. Osteosarcoma
   - _____ D. Chondrosarcoma

2. The large bone forming the heel of the foot is which of the following?
   - _____ A. Talus
   - _____ B. Cuboid
   - _____ C. Navicular
   - _____ D. Calcaneus

3. The flexor tendons extend into the foot anterior or posterior to the ankle joint?
   - _____ A. Anterior
   - _____ B. Posterior

4. The bone that articulates with the three cuneiform bones is which of the following?
   - _____ A. Talus
   - _____ B. Cuboid
   - _____ C. Navicular
   - _____ D. Calcaneus

5. The bone forming the lower end of the ankle joint is which of the following?
   - _____ A. Talus
   - _____ B. Cuboid
   - _____ C. Navicular
   - _____ D. Calcaneus

■ Clinical Case 8-3

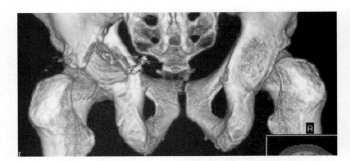 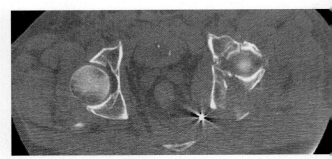

1. Describe the location of the motor vehicle accident (MVA) injury shown in the selected posterior view three-dimensional (3D) and axial computed tomography (CT) images.

   _____

   _____

   _____

2. Describe the changes in adjacent tissues.

   _____

   _____

   _____

3. Describe the consistency, shape, and border.

   _____

   _____

   _____

■ Clinical Case 8-4

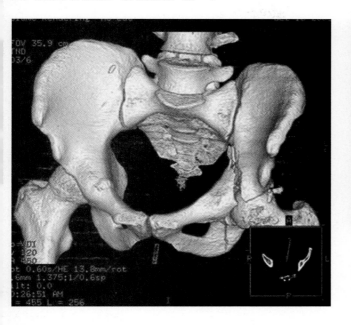

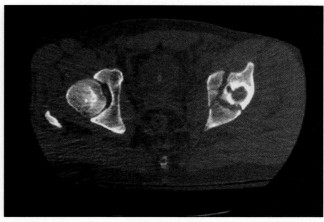

1. Describe the location of the injury in this 26-year-old male patient as shown in the reconstructed anterior view 3D (left) and axial CT (right) images.

   _____

   _____

   _____

2. Describe the changes in adjacent tissues.

   _____

   _____

   _____

3. Describe the consistency, shape, and border.

   _____

   _____

   _____

■ Clinical Case 8-5

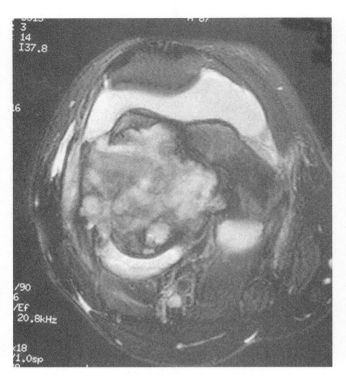 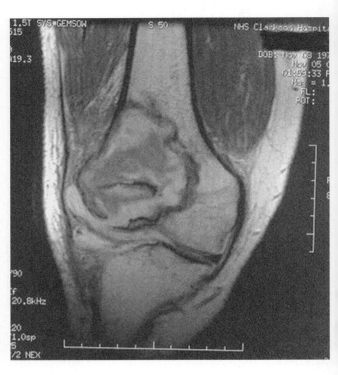

1. Describe the location of the mass discovered in axial (left) and coronal (right) magnetic resonance (MR) images obtained from a 26-year-old man who sustained a knee injury while snowboarding.

   _____

   _____

   _____

2. Describe the changes in adjacent tissues.

   _____

   _____

   _____

3. Describe the consistency, shape, and border.

   _____

   _____

   _____

■ Clinical Case 8-6

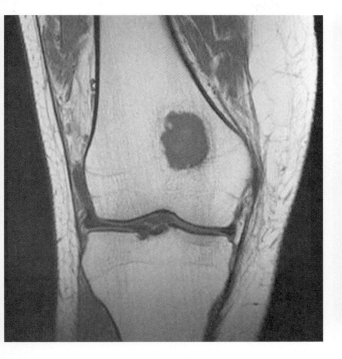
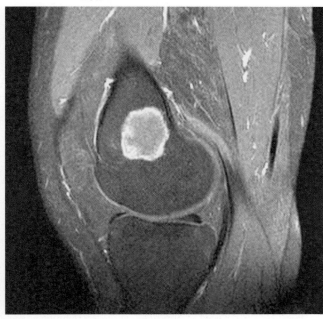

1. Describe the location of the metastatic disease in selected coronal (left) and sagittal (right) MR images of this 23-year-old man previously diagnosed with testicular carcinoma.

   _____

   _____

   _____

2. Describe the changes in adjacent tissues.

   _____

   _____

   _____

3. Describe the consistency, shape, and border.

   _____

   _____

   _____

■ Clinical Case 8-7

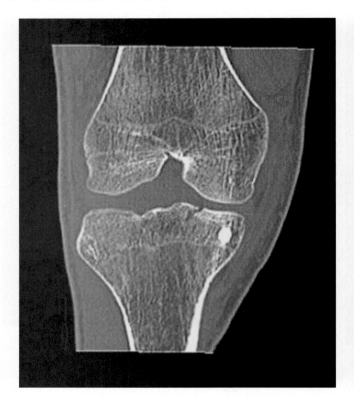 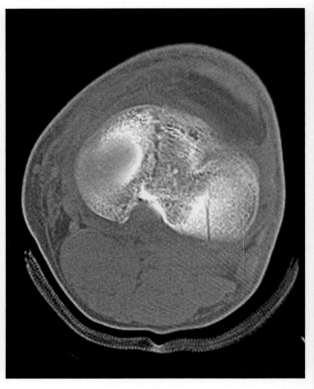

1. Describe the location of the injury in this 28-year-old man shown in the coronal (left) and axial (right) CT images of his right knee. The man presented to the emergency department following MVA.

   _____

   _____

   _____

2. Describe the changes in adjacent tissues.

   _____

   _____

   _____

3. Describe the consistency, shape, and border.

   _____

   _____

   _____

■ Clinical Case 8-8

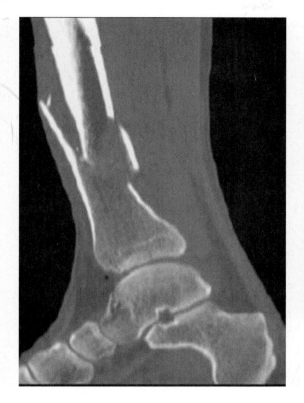
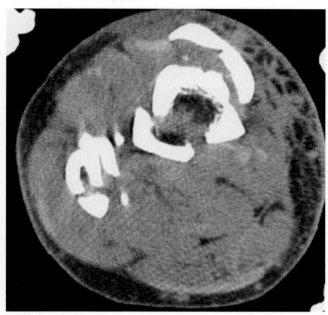

1. Describe the location of the injury as shown in the sagittal (left) and axial (right) CT images.

   _____

   _____

   _____

2. Describe the changes in adjacent tissues.

   _____

   _____

   _____

3. Describe the consistency, shape, and border.

   _____

   _____

   _____